Plastic Surgery

Shehan Hettiaratchy
Matthew Griffiths • Farida Ali
Jon Simmons
(Editors)

Plastic Surgery

A Problem Based Approach

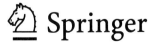 Springer

Editors
Shehan Hettiaratchy, M.A.
(Oxon), BM BCh, FRCS(Eng),
DM, FRCS(Plast)
Department of Plastic
and Reconstructive Surgery
Imperial College Healthcare
NHS Trust, London
UK

Farida Ali, MB ChB, M.Sc.,
FRCS (Plast)
Department of Plastic
and Reconstructive Surgery
St George's Hospital
London, UK

Matthew Griffiths, MBBS, FRCS,
MD, FRCS (Plast)
Department of Plastic
and Reconstructive Surgery
Broomfield Hospital
Chelmsford, UK

Jon Simmons, B.Sc., MBBS,
MRCS, M.Sc. FRCS (Plast)
Department of Plastic
and Reconstructive Surgery
Imperial College Healthcare
NHS Trust, London
UK

ISBN 978-1-84882-115-6   e-ISBN 978-1-84882-116-3
DOI 10.1007/978-1-84882-116-3
Springer London Dordrecht Heidelberg New York

British Library Cataloguing in Publication Data
A catalogue record for this book is available from the British Library

Library of Congress Control Number: 2011933717

Printed on acid-free paper

Springer is part of Springer Science+Business Media (www.springer.com)

Foreword

The surgical trainee is required to assimilate an ever increasing amount of knowledge and for the plastic surgeon this covers a wide area. Consequently, it can sometimes be difficult to maintain attention on the fundamentals of patient assessment. This book aims to bring the focus back on the patient by providing an algorithmic approach to taking a history, examination and formulating a management plan. This refreshingly different clinical problem-based style makes it easy to read. At the end of every chapter the authors provide some key references for further reading.

The book should appeal to the early years trainee as well as to those preparing for clinical examinations

Preface

Plastic surgery is a big subject and the size of traditional text-books reflects this. This book was conceived as something different. Instead of a top-down, subject-by-subject approach, we wanted a bottom-up approach, with the starting point being a patient with a problem. The stimulus for this method was lack of any decent texts for the clinical sections of the professional exams in plastic surgery FRCS Plast in the UK, boards in the USA and their equivalents in other parts of the world). The chapters were written with the concept of a patient sitting in front of the reader, as there would be in the exam situation. However the same approach works when one first sees a patient in the clinic. We aimed to provide the reader with the structure and information necessary to be successful in their careers. We have used our experience to ensure the text is as succinct and relevant as possible. We hope we have achieved this in some way and that this book forms a useful adjunct to more traditional texts.

Many have contributed to the book and we would like to thank them for their hard work and effort. SH would particularly like to thank Jon Simmons for getting us across the finish line; it would not have happened without him and his dogged determination. Finally, we would like to thank our patients from whom we have learnt everything that is in this book.

Shehan Hettiaratchy
Jon Simmons

Acknowledgements

The Editors would specifically like to thank the following for providing the artwork in this book:

Simon Mackey
Specialist Registrar, Plastic and Reconstructive Surgery
Pan-Thames Training Scheme
London, UK

Contents

Contributors

Farida Ali, MB, ChB, MSc, FRCS (Plast)
Department of Plastic and Reconstructive Surgery,
St George's Hospital, London, UK

Robert Caulfield, MB, BCh, BAO (NUI), AFRCSI, MD, FRCSI (Plast)
Specialist Registrar in Plastic and Reconstructive Surgery,
Pan-Thames Training Scheme, London, UK

Matthew Griffiths, MBBS, FRCS, MD, FRCS (Plast)
Department of Plastic and Reconstructive Surgery,
Broomfield Hospital, Chelmsford, UK

Ivo Gwanmesia, BSc, MSc, MBChB, MRCS, FRCS (Plast)
Department of Plastic and Reconstructive Surgery,
Pan-Thames Training Scheme,
London, UK

Fiona Harper, BSc, MBBS, MSc, FRCS (Plast)
Specialist Registrar in Plastic and Reconstructive Surgery,
Pan-Thames Training Scheme,
London, UK

Carolyn Hemsley, MA, (Oxon), PhD, MRCP (UK), FRCPath Directorate of Infections
Guy's and St Thomas' NHS Foundation Trust,
London, UK

John Henton, BSc, MBBS, MRCS (Eng)
Department of Plastic and Reconstructive Surgery,
Imperial College Healthcare NHS Trust, London, UK

**Shehan Hettiaratchy, MA, (Oxon), BM BCh, FRCS (Eng),
DM, FRCS (Plast)** Department of Plastic and
Reconstructive Surgery, Imperial College Healthcare
NHS Trust, London, UK

**Abhilash Jain, MBBS, MRCS (Eng), MSc, PhD,
FRCS (Plast)** Department of Plastic and Reconstructive
Surgery, Imperial College Healthcare NHS Trust London,
London, UK

Jon Simmons, BSc, MBBS, MRCS, MSc, FRCS (Plast)
Department of Plastic and Reconstructive Surgery,
Imperial College Healthcare NHS Trust, London, UK

Abbreviations

a-FP	Alpha-Fetoprotein
ADL	Activities of Daily Living
AP	Antero-Posterior
ATLS	Advanced Trauma Life Support
BAHA	Bone Anchored Hearing Aid
BCC	Basal Cell Carcinoma
BMI	Body Mass Index
BOS	Base of Skull
BPI	Brachial Plexus Injury
BRCA 1/2	Breast Cancer Susceptibility Protein (type 1 or 2)
CMCJ	Carpometacarpal Joint
CP	Cerebral Palsy
CRS	Constriction Ring Syndrome
CSF	Cerebrospinal Fluid
DBUN	Dorsal Branch of Ulnar Nerve
DCIS	Ductal Carcinoma In-Situ
DIC	Disseminated Intravascular Coagulopathy
DIEP	Deep Inferior Epigastric Artery Perforator
DM	Diabetes Mellitus
DN	Digital Nerve
DRUJ	Distal Radio-Ulnar Joint
DVT	Deep Venous Thrombosis
EAM	External Auditory Meatus
ECG	Electro-Cardiograph
EPL	Extensor Policis Longus
FBC	Full Blood Count
FCU	Flexor Carpi Ulnaris

FDP	Flexor Digitorum Profundus
FDS	Flexor Digitorum Superficialis
FHx	Family History
FNA(C)	Fine Needle Aspiration (Cytology)
FPL	Flexor Policis Longus
FSH	Follicle Stimulating Hormone
FTSG	Full Thickness Skin Graft
FTT	Failure to Thrive
g-GT	Gamma-Glytamyl Transpeptidase
GA	General Anaesthetic
GI	Gastro-Intestinal
GnRH	Gonadotropin Releasing Hormone
hCG	Human Chorionic Gonadotropin
HLA	Human Leukocyte Antigen
IDDM	Insulin Dependant Diabetes Mellitus
IGAP	Inferior Gluteal Artery Perforator
IMF	Inframammary Fold
IPJ	Interphalangeal Joint
IVDU	Intravenous Drug User
IVI	Intravenous Infusion
Lat	Lateral
LH	Luteinising Hormone
LMN	Lower Motor Neuron
LS	Lichen Sclerosus
MCN	Musculocutaneous Nerve
MPJ/MCPJ	Metacarpophalangeal Joint
MRD	Marginal Reflex Distance
NAC	Nipple Areolar Complex
NSAID	Non Steroidal Anti Inflammatory Drugs
NVB	Neurovascular Bundle
OPG	Orthopantomogram
ORIF	Open Reduction and Internal Fixation
PCMN	Palmar Cutaneous Branch of Median Nerve
PE	Pulmonary Embolus
PET	Positron Emission Tomography
PIPJ	Proximal Interphalangeal Joint
PIN	Posterior Interosseous Nerve
PVD	Peripheral Vascular Disease

RCT	Randomised Controlled Trial
ROM	Range of Movement
SCC	Squamous Cell Carcinoma
SGAP	Superior Gluteal Artery Perforator
SSG	Split Skin Graft
T4	Thyroxine
TMG	Transverse Myocutaneous Gracilis Flap
TNF	Tumour Necrosis Factor
TOCS	Thoracic Outlet Compression Syndrome
TPF	Temperoparietal Fascia
TRAM	Transverse Rectus Abdominis Myocutaneous
TSH	Thyroid Stimulating Hormone
U+E	Urea and Electrolytes
UCL	Ulnar Collateral Ligament
UMN	Upper Motor Neuron
USS	Ultrasound Scan
VAC	Vacuum Assisted Closure
XR	X-Ray

Chapter 1
Abdominoplasty

Robert Caulfield and Shehan Hettiaratchy

Refers to excision of excess skin and subcutaneous fat from anterior abdominal wall +/– rectus plication.

Recognition

Cosmetic patients are usually female, middle aged, or present post pregnancy with abdominal striae and excess skin. Massive weight loss patients can be either male or female and any age (Fig. 1.1).

History

General introduction
Age, occupation, recent pregnancy/childbirth, interference with lifestyle, relationships, clothing and occupation, diabetes, hypothyroidism.

Specific abdomen
- Is patient's weight stable? (*only operate if weight definitely stable*)
- Have they achieved their target weight/BMI?

R. Caulfield (✉)
Specialist Registrar in Plastic and Reconstructive Surgery,
Pan-Thames Training Scheme,
London, UK

S. Hettiaratchy et al. (eds.), *Plastic Surgery,*
DOI 10.1007/978-1-84882-116-3_1,
© Springer-Verlag London Limited 2012

1

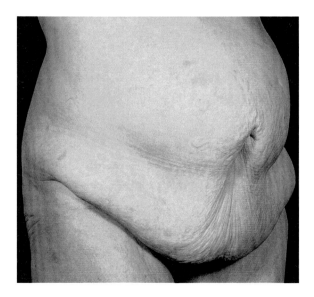

FIGURE 1.1 Pre-operative candidate for abdominoplasty

- Any previous abdominal surgery: Laparoscopy, laparotomy, hernia repair, appendix, open cholecystectomy, hysterectomy, etc.
- Any previous cosmetic abdominal surgery (beware, often these patients will have had previous aesthetic abdominal procedures, e.g., extensive liposuction (implications for blood supply to abdominal pannus) or previous abdominoplasty and will come to clinic with high aesthetic expectations).
- Previous pregnancies, with particular emphasis on whether normal delivery or c-section
- Any current symptoms/signs of abdominal herniae
- Psychological effects of excess abdominal tissue
- Patient's expectations of outcome achieved by surgery
- Awareness of risks and complications associated with surgery

Risk factors

- Multiple previous pregnancies, particularly if more than one c-section (with multiple pregnancies the abdominal wall layers may be very loose/stretched, thus reducing effectiveness and outcome possible with surgery; also risk of bowel/bladder injury with multiple c-sections in the past)
- Previous aesthetic abdominal surgery, particularly extensive liposuction (quite common in these patients, hence risk to blood supply of abdominal pannus)
- Any history of GI or respiratory problems (this can potentially interfere with post-op recovery/mobilisation and increase risk of complications)
- Smoking
- Medication (aspirin, NSAIDs, herbal medications, anticoagulants
- Bleeding tendencies
- Hypertension
- Diabetes
- BMI>30 (known association with increased complications – so used by NHS trusts to rationalise treatment)

General
Full medical and drug history

- Must consider co-existing morbidities relative to risks of procedure (as essentially a cosmetic procedure, in both the pure aesthetic and the massive weight loss cases)
- Family completed or whether planning further children (particularly if you plicate the rectus. Although *Menz, PRS 1996* implies that pregnancy is still possible, but requires close monitoring. Need to discuss this carefully with pre-menopausal female patients pre-op)
- Any psychological issues (i.e., is patient requesting surgery for genuine reasons, as above)
- Occupation and sporting hobbies (as this may interfere with these)

- Any drug allergies
- Medications (as above)
- BMI (weight must be stable)
- Smoking (associated with increased risk of wound break-down/delayed healing)

AIM: By the end of history you should know

1. Extent of patient's symptoms from the excess abdominal pannus
2. Need for additional investigations/ treatment of any co-morbidities prior to GA
3. Patient's awareness of risks/complications
4. What the patient hopes to achieve
5. Chances of surgery meeting these objectives

Examination

Look
Evidence of general obesity. Any overt signs of other significant co-morbidities

- Skin quality and laxity
- Any striae (particularly if supraumbilical, as patient needs to be informed that these will still be present post-op)
- Any scars from previous surgery or c-section. (N.B. make sure to check for very small laparoscopic scars around umbilicus, as these will potentially compromise viability of umbilicus and often patients do not volunteer details about previous laparoscopy – as they consider it a test/ investigation rather than surgery)
- Obvious hernia and bulges
- Whether significant supraumbilical component of excess tissue (i.e., possible Fleur De Lys approach required)

Feel/move
Need to have an idea about the different components of abdominal wall and how you will approach them

- Skin quality and laxity, including scars (both above and below umbilicus)
- Fascial system laxity, i.e., adherence of skin fat to anterior rectus sheath – as this will influence outcome achieved by surgery (both above and below umbilicus)
- Distribution of fat (whether liposuction also required – both above and below umbilicus)
- Tone of abdominal wall, including divarication of recti and any herniae (both above and below umbilicus)

AIM: By the end of examination

1. Identified any previous unknown abdominal pathology which may require investigation/treatment
2. Have decided on most appropriate technique/combination of techniques
3. Have an idea of any problem areas patient wishes to address
4. Awareness of patient's expectations about outcome
5. Willingness of patient to accept downtime and scar maturation period

Investigations

- Routine bloods: FBC, U + E's, Coag, Group and Save
- Depending on co-morbidities, may also need chest X-ray, ECG, etc.

Treatment/Surgical Technique

Depends on examination findings and patient's expectations about outcome, downtime and willingness to accept risks/complications.

Bearing this in mind the surgical options generally depend on the amount each of the different components of abdominal wall are contributing to the overall problem (*Matarasso classification*), as in examination section above. Surgeon preference for scar placement, plication technique and simultaneous liposuction also play a role.

Contribution according to abdominal wall components	Treatment options
Excess fat only	Nothing or liposuction alone
Mild excess skin and fat, no fascial laxity, +/– divarication below umbilicus	Mini-abdominoplasty +/– plication
Moderate excess skin, fat, +/– fascial laxity +/– divarication above and/or below umbilicus	Full abdominoplasty and plication +/– liposuction
Significant excess skin, fat, fascial laxity and divarication	Full abdominoplasty and plication +/– liposuction

Risks/Complications

General

- Risks of GA including DVT/PE/chest infection
- Haematoma
- Drains

Specific

- Wound breakdown/delayed healing
- Decreased or increased sensation in abdominal skin
- Asymmetry, inadequate correction of excess pannus
- Bowel injury (unlikely – but take care when blindly plicating, particularly with round bodied needle)
- Hypertrophic scars (particularly centrally due to excess tension in closure)
- Keloid scars (should avoid these by counselling patient pre-op against surgery)
- Dog ears (particularly laterally – this is often due to deficiencies in pre-op markings, most surgeons will try to address this intra-op with either excision or liposuction)

Post-operative Management

- Expected in-patient stay (2–3 days, but depends on drains)
- Many surgeons advise abdominal binder for the initial post operative period
- Compression garment, such as high cycling shorts for 6 weeks
- Downtime: can be back at sedentary occupation after 2 weeks
- Avoid driving for 2 weeks minimum, even then only short distances for 6 weeks
- Once healed (usually at 2 weeks) can begin massage and moisturisation of scars
- Leave any minor revisions, such as dog ears, for at least 3 months to allow to settle first
- Counsel about duration of 12–18 months for scar maturation

Chapter 2
Blepharoplasty

Robert Caulfield

Refers to adjustment or re-shaping of the appearance of the upper or lower eyelids. Beware the lower lid, skin shortage and ectropion.

Recognition

In the upper lid, patients often present with a degree of cutaneous hooding concealing all or part of the upper eyelid itself in forward gaze. In the lower lid, they present with 'bags', i.e., post-septal fat pads bulging behind a weakened septum. (N.B. Must be aware of co-existing ptosis, as surgical correction is different, as well as any compensated brow ptosis, which may require brow-lifting prior to any upper lid blepharoplasty) (Fig. 2.1).

History

General introduction
Age, occupation, psychological reasons, interference with lifestyle, relationships. General medical conditions such as diabetes and thyroid disease which may also affect the eyes.

R. Caulfield
Specialist Registrar in Plastic and Reconstructive Surgery,
Pan-Thames Training Scheme,
London, UK

S. Hettiaratchy et al. (eds.), *Plastic Surgery*,
DOI 10.1007/978-1-84882-116-3_2,
© Springer-Verlag London Limited 2012

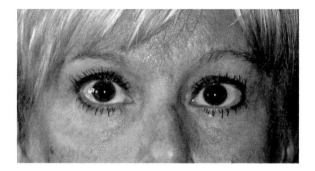

FIGURE 2.1 Pre-operative blepharoplasty candidate

Specific eyes

- Any pre-existing eye disease or defect
- Does the patient wear glasses, contact lenses or combination of both? (N.B. Contact lenses are commonest cause of ptosis in young adults, due to stretching of levator aponeurosis)
- Any history of glaucoma
- Dry eyes
- Excessive tearing (epiphora)
- Redness/soreness
- Double vision (diplopia)
- Any previous aesthetic lid surgery
- Family history: As puffy lower eyelids are often familial and such patients may seek advice at a relatively young age
- Patient's expectations of outcome achieved by surgery
- Awareness of risks and complications associated with surgery

Risk factors

- Any pre-existing eye disease must be documented very clearly pre-op in terms of visual function and fields
- Any significant past medical history of cardiac, GI or respiratory problems (this can potentially interfere with post-op recovery/mobilisation and increase risk of complications)
- Smoking

- Medication (aspirin, NSAIDs, herbal medications, anticoagulants)
- Bleeding tendencies (increased risk of bleeding following post-septal fat excision – risk of retro-orbital haematoma and blindness)
- Hypertension
- Diabetes

General
Full medical and drug history

- Must consider co-existing morbidities relative to risks of procedure (as essentially a cosmetic procedure)
- Full list of medications such as aspirin, NSAIDs, herbal medications, anticoagulants – which can result in catastrophic retro-orbital haematoma (as above)
- Any psychological issues (i.e., is patient requesting surgery for genuine reasons)
- Occupation and sporting hobbies
- Any drug allergies
- Smoking (associated with increased risk of wound breakdown/delayed healing)

AIM: By the end of history you should know

1. Extent of patient's symptoms, e.g., hooding causing interference with visual fields or purely aesthetic reasons
2. Need for additional investigations/treatment of any co-morbidities prior to surgery
3. Patient's awareness of risks/complications
4. What the patient hopes to achieve
5. Chances of surgery meeting these objectives

Examination

Note: Should always have routine assessment by ophthalmologist of patient's visual fields and visual acuity (both with and without glasses and contact lenses) prior to any surgery.

N.B. Patient and examiner should sit opposite each other with their eyes at a similar height and the patient in direct forward gaze.

Look
Eyes

- Any obvious eyelid pathology, e.g., BCCs, SCCs, skin tags, cysts
- Any pre-existing scars
- Skin quality of both upper and lower lids and any wrinkling, particularly at rest
- Orbital asymmetries (dystopia)
- Asymmetries of brow height (brow ptosis – if present will need to be corrected prior to upper lid blepharoplasty, as otherwise will get more noticeable brow ptosis post blepharoplasty)
- Presence of lagophthalmos (inability to close eyes) – if present pre-op, this is an absolute contraindication to aesthetic blepharoplasty
- Position of upper lid (supratarsal) skin crease and any asymmetries between both eyes
- Position of medial and lateral canthi relative to each other
- Any ectropion or entropion
- Any scleral show
- Relationship of globe of eye to orbital margin (vector) – less complications with +ve:
  Negative vector: eye protruding beyond inferior orbital margin
  Positive vector: eye protected by lying behind inferior orbital margin

Feel/move/measure
Examine for brow ptosis, i.e., measure the distance between the mid-pupil and brow apex with callipers: on average is approximately 2.5 cm in adult female. Measure distance from brow apex to anterior frontal hairline: on average is 4.5–6 cm. Thus – if mid-pupil to brow apex height is <2.5 cm and brow apex to hairline height is >6 cm, then you have brow ptosis.

- Check for compensatory brow ptosis, i.e., the brow rises and falls as you open and close the eye.
- Assess for upper lid ptosis: Need to measure MRD1 and MRD2 (marginal reflex distance) and levator function:
    MRD1 = distance from mid-pupillary point to upper lid margin (normal = 5 mm)
    MRD2 = distance from mid-pupillary point to lower lid margin (normal = 5 mm)

Measure levator function (Normal = 15–18 mm)

Subsequent surgical treatment of ptosis depends on amount of ptosis (mild, 1–2 mm; moderate, 2–3 mm; severe, 4 mm or more) and levator function (good if >10 mm and poor if <10 mm).

Assess lower lid laxity and lateral canthal tension using snap test: any delay indicates lack of lower lid support (mandating a transcanthal canthopexy or perhaps canthoplasty).

Location and size of fat pads and degree of prolapse is assessed in both upper and lower lids, simply by gentle pressure on the globe itself.

Assess for presence of Bell's phenomenon, i.e., upward movement of globe on eyelid closure. As absence of Bell's will increase the risk of corneal exposure post-op, particularly if there is any degree of lagophthalmos.

AIM: By the end of the exam

1. Identified any previous unknown eyelid pathology which may require investigation/treatment
2. Determined from ophthalmology report the pre-op status of visual fields and visual acuity
3. Assessed for brow ptosis and compensated brow ptosis
4. Assessed for upper lid ptosis
5. Determined lower lid laxity and lateral canthal tension
6. Confirmed presence of Bell's phenomenon
7. Have decided on most appropriate technique/combination of techniques
8. Have an idea of any problem areas patient wishes to address
9. Awareness of patients expectations about outcome

Investigations

- Opthalmologist assessment of visual fields and visual acuity
- If GA: Routine bloods: FBC, U + E's, Coagulation screen
- If GA and depending on co-morbidities, may also need chest X-ray, ECG etc.

Treatment/Surgical Technique

Depends on examination findings and patient's expectations re outcome, downtime and willingness to accept risks/complications.

Upper lid blepharoplasty:
Can be done under local (infiltration and eye drops) and sedation (much faster recovery and less expensive) or under GA.

Excise skin only first (pinch amount with Adson forceps), then excise partial upper strip of orbicularis (but full width strip laterally – as lateral orbicularis acts as depressor of brow).

Do not disrupt septum or take medial fat pad unless patient specifically requests (while initially looks good, this can hollow when patient ages and there is no way of correcting this).

Lower lid blepharoplasty:
Can be done under local (infiltration and eye drops) and sedation (much faster recovery and less expensive) or under GA.

Always go for transconjunctival approach if possible as much better results (if experienced in the technique) and less complications than subciliary incision.

Transconjunctival: Be careful about removing too much fat. Patients should expect much more conjunctival oedema following this approach.

Transcutaneous/subciliary: Should always simultaneously perform a transcanthal canthopexy to prevent ectropion in immediate post-op period.

Risks/Complications

General

- If under GA include DVT/PE/chest infection

Specific to eye

- Retro-orbital haematoma (rare: approximately 1 in 40,000 if untreated can cause blindness)
- Ectropion, i.e., resulting from overcorrection with lower lid blepharoplasty (avoid by taking minimal amount of lower lid skin and always performing transcanthal canthopexy)
- Excessive scleral show (again avoid in same way as for ectropion)
- Over-correction with upper lid blepharoplasty resulting in lagophthalmos (always store the excised skin, but be aware of Human Tissue Act in this regard)
- Under-correction with upper lid blepharoplasty with residual hooding
- Under-correction with lower lid blepharoplasty fat excision with residual prominent 'bags'
- Corneal abrasions (treat with contact lens dressing for 5–7 days)

Post-operative Management

- If done under local and sedation, then can go home same day
- Avoid any strenuous activity, heavy lifting, sports for minimum of 2 weeks
- Downtime: can be back at sedentary occupation after 2 weeks
- Sutures out at 5 days
- Warn about appearance of elevated lateral canthus if transcanthal canthopexy performed along with lower lid blepharoplasty
- Counsel about duration of 12–18 months for scar maturation

Anatomy of the Lids (*Fig. 2.2*)

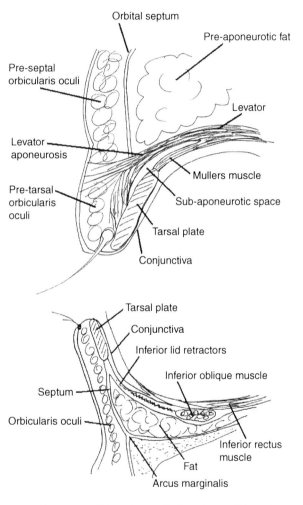

FIGURE 2.2 *Top*: upper lid anatomy, *Bottom*: lower lid anatomy

Chapter 3
Breast Reconstruction

Robert Caulfield and Matthew Griffiths

Occurs most commonly as either immediate or delayed reconstruction following mastectomy +/– axillary dissection. Recently, oncoplastic techniques are being used to optimise aesthetic results following wide local excision of breast lumps.

Recognition

Often in combination with general/breast surgeons in joint clinics prior to tumour removal or following referral from them for either immediate or delayed reconstruction. Type and extent of reconstruction depends on tumour treatment (particularly adjuvant therapy such as radiotherapy), patient choice/expectations and experience/capability of reconstructive team (Fig. 3.1).

R. Caulfield (✉)
Specialist Registrar in Plastic and Reconstructive Surgery,
Pan-Thames Training Scheme,
London, UK

S. Hettiaratchy et al. (eds.), *Plastic Surgery*,
DOI 10.1007/978-1-84882-116-3_3,
© Springer-Verlag London Limited 2012

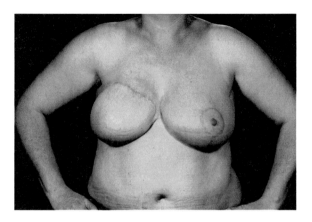

FIGURE. 3.1 Patient post DIEP breast reconstruction pre-symmetrization

History

General

Age, occupation, recent pregnancy/childbirth/family completed. Detailed past medical history (as co-morbidities will impact significantly on choice of reconstruction), social history, medications and smoking.

Specific breast cancer

- Family history of breast cancer
- Any genetic high risk, e.g., BRCA1 or BRAC2
- Personal history of previous/current lumps, nipple discharge, skin retraction, inverted nipples
- Any previous breast investigations and the results
- Any pre-op therapy planned, e.g., chemotherapy
- Surgical management plan by general breast surgeons
- Post-op adjuvant therapy planned, e.g., radiotherapy or chemotherapy (Must be aware of exact timings)

Risk factors

- Tumour grade/extent/stage
- Age: may influence reconstructive options

- Multiple co-morbidities
- General obesity: Will be associated with significant increase of complications
- Family history of breast cancer (as above)
- Smoking: Associated with wound healing problems, poor vessels/blood flow in free flaps and increase in anaesthetic related complications, e.g., chest infection, DVT PE
- Medication (aspirin, NSAIDs, herbal medications, anticoagulants)
- Bleeding tendencies
- Hypertension
- Diabetes
- BMI >30

Breast reconstruction history

- Current breast size/shape
- Patient desire for post-op size/shape
- Patient's awareness of reconstructive options and specific requests for particular reconstruction
- Patient willingness to have symmetrisation procedures on the other side
- Past surgical history, particularly abdominal surgery (be aware that increasingly units are being more expansive in their approach to such cases and often they can be considered as relative contraindications or considered as 'more complex' rather than absolute contraindications)
- Patient's weight stable (as otherwise DIEP/TRAM reconstruction will change as weight changes)
- Patient's occupation, hobbies, sports
- Acceptance of donor site morbidity and outcome

AIM: by the end of history you should know

1. Patient's expected treatment plan
2. Tumour related factors that may influence type of reconstruction
3. Patient related factors that may influence type of reconstruction
4. Patient's choice/request for specific reconstruction

5. Patient awareness of reconstructive pathway, risks/complications, duration and timing
6. Chances of reconstructive surgery meeting patient's objectives

Examination

Look
Evidence of general obesity, any overt signs of other significant co-morbidities.

Breast
Cancer exam first
In immediate cases, will already be well documented by general breast surgeon, but will help in planning size, shape and inset of flap/reconstruction.

In delayed cases, will identify any previously unknown problems on unaffected side, as well as assisting in planning size, shape and inset of flap/reconstruction

- Look for symmetry (immediate cases), lumps, skin retraction, inverted nipples, nipple discharge
- Examine standing or sitting up: first arms by side, then on hips flexing pectoralis major and then arms above head
- Examine both breasts for abnormal lumps (NAC, four quadrants and tail of breast) with patient lying down and arm above head for each side
- Examine both axillae for any nodes

Aesthetic exam

- Examine with patient standing up, looking straight ahead and hands on hips
- In delayed cases, examine with bra on, as this allows you to gauge volume/size of reconstruction required (particularly if patient does not want any symmetrisation on normal side post-op)
- In delayed cases: need to assess volume of tissue required and amount of skin and ptosis required to match opposite side

- Assess suitability of opposite side for subsequent masto-pexy/reduction procedure
- Measure sternal notch to nipple distance and nipple to IMF on normal side and correlate with ideal position on side to be reconstructed
- Skin quality (particularly if previous radiotherapy and if previous smoker or other co-morbidities)
- Presence of any scars

Abdomen (DIEP/TRAM donor site)

- Extent of available abdominal pannus
- Presence of divarication of recti or any hernia
- Any abdominal scars, e.g., appendix, laparoscopy, laparo-tomy, c-section/pfannenstiel, hysterectomy, Kocher's, etc. (as noted in breast reconstruction history – are now considered more complex cases or relative contraindications, rather than absolute contraindications)

Back (latissimus dorsi donor site)

- Presence or absence of lat. dorsi (N.B. Poland's syndrome)
- Volume of adipose tissue
- Amount of excess skin
- Presence of pre-existing scars

Thigh (TMG donor site)

- Volume of adipose tissue
- Amount of excess skin
- Presence of pre-existing scars

Buttock (SGAP/IGAP donor site)

- Volume of adipose tissue
- Amount of excess skin
- Presence of pre-existing scars

AIM: by the end of exam

1. Identified most appropriate donor site for reconstruction
2. Have secondary 'back-up' donor in case of problems with first choice
3. Have an idea of any problem areas patient wishes to address

4. Awareness of patient's expectations about outcome and reconstruction pathway
5. Willingness of patient to accept downtime and subsequent symmetrisation and adjustment phase of reconstruction

Investigations

Routine bloods: FBC, U + E's, coag, group and crossmatch
CT angiogram (not routine in every unit, but increasingly used to plan pre-op for DIEPs).

Additional radiological/cytological/histological investigations *only if clinical suspicion:*

- Radiology: Ultrasound breast (if < 35 years old)
- Mammogram breast (if > 35 years old and suspicious lump or if > 50 years old and > 1 year since last mammogram)
- Ultrasound axillae (if palpable axillary nodes)
- Cytology/Histology: i.e., FNA or Trucut biopsy of suspicious lumps or nodes

Treatment/Surgical Technique

Depends if immediate or delayed reconstruction, any pre-op therapy, post-op radiotherapy/chemotherapy, as well as examination findings, suitable donors to provide optimal reconstruction and patient's expectations.

Ultimately tumour treatment and patient survival is most important, so reconstruction should not interfere in any way with this. Remember low grade DCIS patients can survive for a long time, and high grade tumours often have limited prognosis (so simpler, less complicated reconstructions may be more appropriate).

Considering all of the above, rigid reconstruction rules do not apply (apart from avoiding implant based reconstructions if post-op radiotherapy is planned). So any reconstruction can be any one or combination of those below.

Note: Autologous reconstructions can include:
Extended Lat Dorsi, DIEP/TRAM, SGAP/IGAP, TMG.

An example of a reasonable general approach and options for reconstruction:

	Young, fit and well	Radiotherapy	Old and infirm
Small breast	1. Expander 2. Lat. dorsi and implant 3. Autologous	1. Autologous	1. Expander 2. Lat. dorsi and implant
Moderate breast	1. Expander and mastopexy/ reduction 2. Lat. dorsi and implant and mastopexy/ reduction 3. Autologous	1. Autologous	1. Expander
Large breast	1. Nothing 2. Expander and reduction 3. Lat. dorsi and implant and reduction 4. Autologous	1. Nothing 2. Lat. dorsi and implant and reduction 3. Autologous	1. Nothing 2. Expander and reduction

Risks/Complications

General

- Risks of GA including DVT/PE/Chest infection
- Haematoma
- Drains

Specific

Flap problems:

- Flap loss/failure
- Partial flap loss/fat necrosis
- Delayed wound healing/wound breakdown (can delay start of adjuvant therapy)

Donor problems:

- Haematoma
- Hernia/bowel injury (with DIEP/TRAM – but very low risk with modern techniques)
- Delayed wound healing/wound breakdown (can delay start of adjuvant therapy)

Implant/expander problems:

- Haematoma
- Infection
- Extrusion
- Delayed wound healing/wound breakdown (can delay start of adjuvant therapy)
- Capsular contraction and pain

Post-operative Management

Depends on:

- Type of reconstruction performed
- Immediate post-op complications
- Unit protocol for post-op care and discharge of flap reconstructions
- Timing of any planned adjuvant therapy

Chapter 4
Large Breasts/Reduction

Robert Caulfield and Matthew Griffiths

Bilateral mammary hypertrophy/hyperplasia. Often asymmetrical. Can also be associated with significant ptosis – so be aware of overlap of reduction approach/techniques with mastopexy approach/techniques.

Recognition

Can present at any age post puberty: But usually young females in early 20s or women in 40s after completion of family. Recognise by excess of breast tissue +/– excess skin, +/– ptosis, combined with presenting symptoms (see below) (Fig. 4.1).

History

General introduction
Age, symptoms and duration, occupation, N.B. interference with lifestyle, relationships, clothing and occupation. Neck pain and shoulder pain (N.B. warn patients that neck/shoulder pain may be due to other causes and may not resolve post-op). Diabetes, hypothyroidism.

R. Caulfield (✉)
Specialist Registrar in Plastic and Reconstructive Surgery,
Pan-Thames Training Scheme,
London, UK

S. Hettiaratchy et al. (eds.), *Plastic Surgery*,
DOI 10.1007/978-1-84882-116-3_4,
© Springer-Verlag London Limited 2012

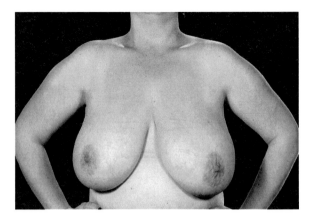

FIGURE 4.1 Candidate for breast reduction

Specific breast

- Grooving
- Intertrigo/maceration
- Requirement to wear bra at night
- Psychological effects
- Pain (Must make sure patient is wearing correct bra size (see below) – commonest cause of breast pain)
- Family history of breast cancer
- Personal history of previous/current lumps, discharge, skin retraction, inverted nipples
- Any previous breast investigations and the results: FNAs, biopsies, ultrasound, mammogram

Risk factors

- Family history of breast cancer
- General obesity: In younger women – associated with oestrogen induced increase in dense glandular tissue; in older women – associated with increase in fatty/adipose content of breast
- Smoking
- Medication
- Bleeding tendencies

- Hypertension
- Diabetes
- BMI>30 (known association with increased complications – so used by NHS trusts to rationalise treatment)

General
Full medical and drug history

- Must consider co-morbidities in risk/benefit analysis
- Family completed or whether planning further children (implications for breast feeding)
- Any psychological issues (i.e. is patient requesting surgery for genuine reasons)
- Any drug allergies
- Medications (as above)
- BMI (weight must be stable)
- Smoking (associated with increased risk of wound breakdown/delayed healing)

AIM: by the end of history you should know

1. Extent of patient's symptoms
2. Need for additional investigations/treatment of any intrinsic breast lump/problem
3. Patient's awareness of risks and complications
4. What the patient hopes to achieve
5. Chances of surgery meeting these expectations

Examination

Look
Evidence of general obesity. Any overt signs of other significant co-morbidities.

Breast – cancer exam first

- Look for symmetry, lumps, skin retraction, inverted nipples, nipple discharge
- Examine standing or sitting up: first arms by side, then on hips flexing pec. major and then arms above head

- Examine both breasts for abnormal lumps (NAC, four quadrants and tail of breast) with patient lying down and arm above head for each side
- Examine both axillae for any nodes

Aesthetic breast exam

- Initially examine with bra on: to determine if correct size/ possible cause of breast pain (particularly if pain is the patient's main reason for requesting a reduction)
- Examine with patient standing up, looking straight ahead and hands on hips
- Assess approximate cup size and asymmetry:

Measure chest circumference at IMF level:

If even number: add 4 in. This gives the bra size
If odd number: add 5 in. i.e., 34 or 36 etc.

Measure breast circumference at most prominent part of breast:

If equal to IMF measurement – then AA cup
If 2 cm (1 in.) more – then A cup
If 4 cm (2 in.) more – then B cup etc.

- Grade of ptosis (see mastopexy chapter)
- Measure sternal notch to nipple distance
- Measure nipple to IMF distance
- Inspect for stretch marks
- Skin quality
- Presence of any scars: N.B. previous wide local excision for breast lump (will need to consider altering skin excision technique to possibly include scar); previous duct excision for benign nipple discharge (will have partial periareolar scar, but significant risk to nipple viability if pedicle is based in same area, so will need to change location of dermoglandular pedicle).

AIM: by the end of exam

1. Identifyied any previous unknown breast pathology
2. Have an idea of any problem areas patient wishes to address

3. Have decided on most appropriate technique
4. Awareness of patient's expectations
5. Willingness of patient to accept downtime and scar maturation period

Investigations

- Routine bloods: FBC, U + E's, coag
- Cytology/Histology: i.e. FNA or Trucut biopsy of suspicious lumps or nodes
- Additional radiological/cytological/histological investigations *only if clinical suspicion:*
    - Radiology: Ultrasound breast (if < 35 years old)
    - Mammogram breast (if > 35 years old and suspicious lump or if > 50 years old and >1 year since last mammogram)
    - Ultrasound axillae (if palpable axillary nodes)

Treatment/Surgical Technique

Depends on examination findings and patient's expectations about outcome and willingness to accept risks/complications:

- Amount of expected tissue to be resected from each side:
- 32–34 in. chest – one cup size = 100 g
- 36 in. chest or > – one cup size = 180–200 g
- Skin quality and amount of excess skin
- Degree of ptosis
- Nipple to IMF distance
- Patient's age: younger patient's skin more elastic (better results with vertical scar than older patient)
- Smoker/ex-smoker/non-smoker

Technique
All based on dermoglandular pedicle: Can be inferior, superomedial or central superior depending on surgeon's preference and experience.

Some general guidelines (but considerable variation in approach depending on surgeon's preference and experience):

1. Very small reduction: Liposuction only. Easier in older atrophic, less glandular breasts
2. Ptosis only: Mastopexy technique (see mastopexy chapter)
3. Sternal notch to nipple distance:
   - Less than 30 cm   Vertical scar technique (but only if young, good quality elastic skin and non-smoker)
   - Greater than 30 cm   Wise pattern technique of your choice
   - Greater than 40 cm   Warn of risk of free nipple graft

Risks/Complications

General

- Risks of GA including DVT/PE/Chest infection
- Haematoma

Specific
Nipples:

- Nipple loss/necrosis (partial or complete)
- Decreased or increased sensation
- De-pigmentation of NAC

Wound:

- Delayed healing
- T junction breakdown

Scar:

- Hypertrophic scars (particularly at medial and lateral extent of wounds)
- Keloid scars (very important to counsel at risk patients adequately pre-operatively)
- Dog ears (particularly laterally – this is often due to deficiencies in pre-op markings)

Gland:

- Loss of ability to breastfeed (should have identified preoperatively whether family complete; however up to 70% can still lactate post-op)
- Residual asymmetry

Post-operative Management

- Expected in-patient stay (1–3 days, but depends on drains – a lot of surgeons routinely do *not* use drains with reductions anymore, so can often discharge day after surgery)
- Downtime: can be back at sedentary occupation within 2 weeks
- Avoid driving for 2 weeks
- Wear sports bra day and night for 6 weeks
- Once healed (usually at 2 weeks) can begin massage and moisturisation of scars
- Counsel about duration of 12–18 months for scar maturation

Chapter 5
Ptotic Breasts/Mastopexy

Robert Caulfield and Matthew Griffiths

Pure ptosis refers to descent of NAC and breast tissue below the IMF (see grading below). Often asymmetrical. Often associated with mammary hypertrophy/hyperplasia – so be aware of overlap of mastopexy approach/techniques with reduction approach/techniques.

Recognition

Usually patients present post childbirth with post-pregnancy involutional changes, volume loss, striae, etc. (N.B. These cases often require augment-mastopexy approach; assess very carefully pre-op) But usually women in 40s or older with moderate ptosis. Often associated with excess breast tissue and asymmetrical, so take care to assess in detail pre-op about all aspects, i.e., skin, breast, NAC and most importantly patient's expectations about outcome (Fig. 5.1).

R. Caulfield (✉)
Specialist Registrar in Plastic and Reconstructive Surgery,
Pan-Thames Training Scheme,
London, UK

S. Hettiaratchy et al. (eds.), *Plastic Surgery*,
DOI 10.1007/978-1-84882-116-3_5,
© Springer-Verlag London Limited 2012

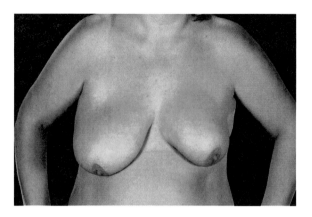

FIGURE 5.1 Patient with ptotic breasts

History

General introduction
Age, duration of problem and symptoms, occupation, recent pregnancy/childbirth, is family complete, interference with lifestyle, relationships, clothing and occupation, diabetes, hypothyroidism. (Neck pain and shoulder pain are usually not an issue in pure mastopexy cases, unless associated with significant mammary hypertrophy/hyperplasia).

Specific: Breast

- Recent changes in bra size (hence breast volume)
- Any previous aesthetic breast surgery (these patients often have high aesthetic expectations – must know details of surgery)
- Grooving
- Intertrigo/maceration
- Requirement to wear bra at night
- Psychological effects
- Pain (must make sure patient is wearing correct bra size – commonest cause of breast pain)
- Family history of breast cancer
- Personal history of previous/current lumps, discharge, skin retraction, inverted nipples
- Any previous breast investigations and the results: FNAs, biopsies, ultrasound, mammogram

Risk factors

- Multiple previous pregnancies (hence significant involutional volume loss and striae, poor skin quality)
- Previous aesthetic breast surgery (see above)
- General obesity in younger women, much denser breast, hence get good results with mastopexy alone, often vertical scar possible
- General obesity in older women, more fatty breast and less easy to get good projection, so often require augment-mastopexy).
- Family history of breast cancer
- Smoking
- Medication
- Bleeding tendencies
- Hypertension
- Diabetes
- BMI > 30 (known association with increased complications – so used by NHS trusts to rationalise treatment)

General

Full medical and drug history

- Must consider co-existing morbidities relative to risks of procedure (as essentially a cosmetic procedure)
- Family completed or whether planning further kids (implications for breast feeding and postpartum shape/volume changes)
- Any psychological issues (i.e., is patient requesting surgery for genuine reasons, as above)
- If augment-mastopexy required, does patient wish for one stage procedure, or happy to have two stage (implications for cost (if private) and also downtime. Also awareness of future implant related ops.
- Any drug allergies
- Medications (as above)
- BMI (weight must be stable)
- Smoking (associated with increased risk of wound breakdown/delayed healing)

AIM: by the end of history you should know

1. Extent of patient's symptoms
2. Need for additional investigations/treatment of any intrinsic breast lump/problem

3. Patient's awareness of risks/complications
4. What the patient hopes to achieve
5. One stage or two stage preferred by surgeon and/or by patient
6. Chances of surgery meeting these objectives

Examination

Look
Evidence of general obesity. Any overt signs of other significant co-morbidities.

Breast
Cancer exam first

- Look for symmetry, lumps, skin retraction, inverted nipples, nipple discharge
- Examine standing or sitting up: first arms by side, then on hips flexing pec major and then arms above head
- Examine both breasts for abnormal lumps (NAC, four quadrants and tail of breast) with patient lying down and arm above head for each side
- Examine both axillae for any nodes

Aesthetic exam

- Initially examine with bra on: to determine if correct size-possible cause of breast pain
- Examine with patient standing up, looking straight ahead and hands on hips
- Particularly important to assess upper pole breast volume – pinch test:
  If > 2 in. breast tissue upper pole can go subglandular
  If < 2 in. breast tissue upper pole must go submuscular
- Assess grade of ptosis (Regnault):
  - Normal breast: NAC above IMF, breast tissue at or above IMF
  - Grade 1: Nipple at IMF and above most dependent breast tissue

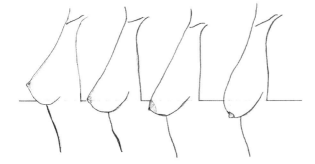

FIGURE 5.2 Grades 1–3 ptosis

- Grade 2: Top of NAC at IMF and above most dependent breast tissue
- Grade 3: NAC below IMF and below most dependent breast tissue
- Pseudoptosis: NAC above IMF, but breast tissue below IMF (usually post reduction) (Fig. 5.2)
- Measure sternal notch to nipple distance
- Measure nipple to IMF distance
- Stretch marks/striae
- Skin quality (particularly if previous smoker or other co-morbidities)
- Presence of any scars

AIM: by the end of exam

1. Identified any previous unknown breast pathology/suspected cancer which may require investigation/treatment
2. Have decided on most appropriate technique/combination of techniques
3. If augment-mastopexy required: whether one stage or two stage (surgeon preference versus patient preference)
4. Have an idea of any problem areas patient wishes to address
5. Awareness of patient's expectations about outcome

Investigations

- Routine bloods: FBC, U + E's
- Additional radiological/cytological/histological investigations *only if clinical suspicion.*

Treatment/Surgical Technique

Depends on examination findings and patient's expectations about outcome, downtime and willingness to accept risks/complications.

- If mastopexy alone, which skin excision technique will give best results in terms of breast tissue re-modelling, as well as most appropriate skin resection to give optimum projection and shape
- If augment-mastopexy, whether one stage or two stage and how to manage patient's expectations about results and downtime, particularly if two stage approach

Technique

As described above, technique can be mastopexy alone, or augment-mastopexy, which can in turn be one or two stages (if two stages should do augment first, followed by mastopexy a minimum of 3 months later).

Mastopexy alone techniques:
All based on same approach taken to reduction cases.

Skin excision:

- Periareolar: but take care, these scars can stretch badly and often leave visible white scar as result
- Vertical scar: Rule of thumb, only if young, good elastic skin quality, non-smoker and only need to lift nipple less than 10 cm, i.e., most tend to be grade 1 or 2 ptosis
- Wise pattern: Tend to need in most cases, as the self-selecting patient population are older, poor skin quality, often smokers/ex-smokers, and anyone with grade 3 ptosis

Breast tissue re-modelling:
Use a dermoglandular pedicle (as with reduction cases), which can be inferior, superomedial or central superior depending on surgeon's preference and experience. Rather than excise tissue (unless needed), you simply re-position/re-mould tissue to give ideal projection and shape.

Augment-mastopexy techniques:
As noted above, can be one or two stage

If one stage:

- Do augment first (either subglandular or submuscular – see 'Examination' section)
- Then mastopexy, using most appropriate combination of skin excision and breast re-modelling techniques as above

If two stage:

- Same approach as one stage, except separate by 3 months, which allows the subsequent mastopexy to be more effective (but must carefully manage patient's expectations).

Risks/Complications

General

- Risks of GA: DVT/PE/chest infection
- Haematoma
- Drains (often not used in pure mastopexy cases)

Specific
Nipples:

- Nipple loss/necrosis (partial or complete – again less likely than in reduction cases)
- Decreased or increased sensation
- Depigmentation of NAC

Wound:

- Delayed healing
- T junction breakdown

Scar:

- Hypertrophic scars (particularly at medial and lateral extent of wound)
- Keloid scars (Ensure susceptible patients are properly counselled about the potential risks)
- Dog ears (particularly laterally)

Gland:

- Lack of projection
- Insufficient volume in upper pole
- Loss of ability to breastfeed (Patients should be counselled about this pre-operatively if family incomplete - approximately 70% can still lactate post-op)
- Residual asymmetry

Post-operative Management

- Expected in-patient stay (2–3 days, but depends on drains – a lot of surgeons routinely do *not* use drains anymore, so can often discharge day after surgery)
- Downtime: can be back at sedentary occupation within 2 weeks
- Avoid driving for 2 weeks
- Wear sports bra day and night for 6 weeks
- Once healed (usually at 2 weeks) can begin massage and moisturising scars
- If two stage augment-mastopexy, counsel about expectations after first op (augment) and need for 3 month delay before second stage
- Counsel about duration of 12–18 months for scar maturation

Chapter 6
Burns Contracture

Farida Ali and Jon Simmons

Prevention is better than cure. Children, in particular, who have sustained burns should be followed up regularly to allow early identification of problematic scars.

Recognition

Burn scar contracture can result in both functional and aesthetic problems. The aim of treatment should firstly be to improve function, particularly in vital areas such as periorbital, hand or perioral (Fig. 6.1).

History

General introduction
Age, occupation, handedness, interference with lifestyle, relationships, smoking and occupation. Co-morbidities and medication.

F. Ali (✉)
Department of Plastic and Reconstructive Surgery,
St George's Hospital,
London, UK

S. Hettiaratchy et al. (eds.), *Plastic Surgery*,
DOI 10.1007/978-1-84882-116-3_6,
© Springer-Verlag London Limited 2012

41

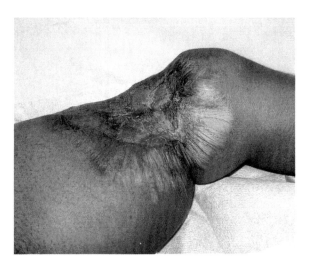

FIGURE 6.1 Burn contracture

Specific burn history

- Mechanism of burn
- How long ago
- Initial treatment
- Time to healing (>3/52 higher risk of problematic scars)
- Complications such as infection
- Length of time in hospital: to give an idea of the complexity of the burn

Define the problem

- What is the patient's assessment of any problems
- Unstable skin, ulceration and bleeding, pain and itching
- Facial: asymmetry, scarring, think about cosmetic units
- Periorbital scars: eye opening or closure, watering
- Perioral scars: microsomia, inability to close mouth?
- Neck: restricted range of movement. Does it pull down/distort the mouth upon movement?

- Breast: abnormal breast development (especially with burns sustained in prepubertal girls)?
- Joints
  - Axillary contracture. Limitation of arm and shoulder movement? Ask about any difficulty dressing (doing up a bra, fastening buttons), personal care, e.g., brushing hair
  - Popliteal fossa: limited leg extension? Difficulty walking?
  - Feet: hyperextension of the toes – problems with footwear?
  - Hands: Is the wrist affected? Limitation of finger extension more common. Can prevent or restrict coarse and fine grip

AIM: by the end of the history you should

1. Have a full understanding of the history of the burn and its cause and initial treatment
2. Understand how long different areas of the burn took to heal and any complications
3. Have a thorough understanding of the patient's functional level
4. Understand what the patient hopes to achieve from any further treatment
5. Know any factors which might influence treatment: co-morbidities, occupation, etc.

Examination

Look

- Assess the patient's skin from head to toe, then concentrate on the problem areas
- Where is it?
- Does it cross joints or cosmetic units?

- Is there distortion at rest?
- What is the morphology of the burn: linear scar or large confluence?
- Is the scar mature or immature, keloid or hypertrophic?
- What is the quality of the burn tissue and surrounding tissues?

Move

- Take the patient through the range of movement specific to that area.
- Note any limitation in movement and distortion of neighbouring structures as they go through their range of motion.
- Ask the patient to perform simple activities that demonstrate the degree (and impact) of such limitation.
    - Put your chin on your chest
    - Look up to the ceiling
    - Look over your left/right shoulder
    - Close your eyes
    - Smile
    - Close your mouth (with and without neck extension)
    - Put your hands behind your head/back
    - Lift your arms above your head
    - Straighten your arm
    - Put your hands flat on the table
    - Make a fist
- Ask them to walk noting any deviation from the normal gait cycle.
- Examine the neighbouring tissues to evaluate the potential use in the reconstructive options.

AIM: by the end of the examination you should

1. Understand any functional or cosmetic implications of the burn
2. Have assessed surrounding tissues for local treatment options

3. Have assessed remote sites for potential donor sites
4. Have formulated some plans for treatment

Investigations

- Routine bloods: FBC, U + E's, Coagulation, Group and Save
- Depending on co-morbidities, may also need chest X-ray, ECG etc.
- If joints are involved, relevant x-rays

Treatment

Early

- Pressure therapy: need to work closely with the OT who need to ensure the pressure garment fits well and is changed as necessary to allow growth
- Splint: Resting and night splints to prevent/minimise deformity
- Physiotherapy: to preserve as much range of motion as possible
- Surgery rarely indicated but may be required to protect eye

Surgical treatment is usually only considered in mature scars.
  Local flaps: The use of local flaps alone requires adequate tissue laxity in the surrounding skin and soft tissue

- Z plasty
- Y–V flaps

Tissue expansion

- With second stage local flap (advancement, transposition, rotation)
- Beware the lower limb where expansion is fraught with difficulties

Resurfacing

- FTSG: better than STSG because of less contraction and better colour match. Maybe useful in burn contractures of the neck. Not so useful in contractures around joints, which require durable tissue.
- Distant flap: includes fasciocutaneous and musculocutaneous flaps, e.g., latissimus dorsi flap for axillary scar release, TFL flap for groin
- Free flaps
- Skin substitutes

Chapter 7
Burns

Farida Ali, Abhilash Jain, and Jon Simmons

As with all trauma, burns patients should be managed according to ATLS guidelines. Types: minor, major and burns in special sites.

Recognition

Establish the history early as facial and/or airway swelling may make this difficult later on. Flame burns and chemical burns are most common in adults. In children and the elderly, scalds are more common. For this group, non-accidental injury must also be considered.

Referral to a burns unit
National Burn Care Review Group guidelines:

- Major burns (>10% in children, >20% in adults)
- Full thickness burns >5% TBSA
- Inhalational injury
- Specific mechanisms (chemical burns (esp. hydrofluoric acid), high tension electrical burns)
- Special sites (facial, hands, feet, perineum, flexor surfaces, circumferential burns)

F. Ali (✉)
Department of Plastic and Reconstructive Surgery,
St George's Hospital,
London, UK

S. Hettiaratchy et al. (eds.), *Plastic Surgery*,
DOI 10.1007/978-1-84882-116-3_7,
© Springer-Verlag London Limited 2012

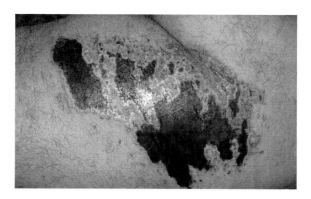

FIGURE 7.1 Acute chemical burn

- Special groups (the elderly (>60), very young (<5), NAI)
- Concomitant injury/coexisting disease (Fig. 7.1)

History

Specific
The type of burn:

- Flame: flash burn, explosion, clothes on fire, extinguished, enclosed space, first aid measures
- Scalds: immersion or spill, source (boiled water, with or without milk, other (e.g., oil – deeper burns), bath water)
- Electrical: high tension or domestic, lightening strike, arcing, collapse (cardiac arrest/arrhythmia), contact time
- Chemical: acid or alkali, time of exposure, irrigation, neutralisation
- Contact: temperature, industrial (much higher temperatures) versus domestic

Respiratory complications: 10–20% of patients admitted for major burns have an associated inhalational injury. Consider the possibility of direct injury to the airways, smoke inhalation, blast injury (mechanical trauma to the lungs/alveolae, ARDS).

The timings:

Time of burn itself
Exposure time

Time first aid measures commenced
Length of time of cooling/irrigation
Time fluids started (if any)

Circumstances of burn:
Accidental, non-accidental, self-inflicted? Self-inflicted injuries often obvious. Non-accidental injuries (NAI) however can be difficult to identify but are extremely important to recognise. Consider in all burns in children and the elderly. Check 'at risk' register. If any suggestion of NAI, child protection services need to be involved. Although distressing for the family, primary concern is patient safety. Suspect if any of the following are present:

- Delayed presentation
- Changing history
- History/signs of previous injuries of varying age
- Inappropriate reactions (over the top or no interest)
- Inappropriate interaction between involved parties

Concomitant injuries:
Did they need to jump out of a building? Was there an explosion? With high-tension electrical injuries, patients can be thrown a significant distance, sustaining mechanical trauma in addition to the burn injury. Blast injury?

Other:
Co-morbidities/smoker? This will affect the carboxyhaemoglobin result.
Drug history/allergies

Examination

As per ATLS guidelines
Airway (with Cx Spine control):
If conscious, is the patient talking? Airway burns are those above the level of the vocal cords. Facial/oral/mucosal burns/oedema. Singeing of nasal hairs. Carbonaceous sputum. Stridor. Hoarse voice.

Breathing (with 100% oxygen via a non-rebreather bag):
Signs include: tachypnoea, dyspnoea. Abnormal chest movements (circumferential deep dermal/full thickness burns of the torso or associated mechanical trauma). Crepitations. Pulmonary oedema. Signs of ARDS. Reduced oxygen saturations (may be falsely high in carboxyhaemoglobin toxicity). Arterial blood gas analysis may reveal hypoxia or raised carboxyhaemoglobin (>25–30% in a non-smoker is an indication for ventilation).

ANY concerns about actual or potential airway or breathing complications should initiate anaesthetic input to assess the patient, securing a protected airway and providing respiratory support where indicated. Intubation is indicated in all patients prior to transfer to a burns unit where there is potential for respiratory compromise, irrespective of whether they show signs or not at the referring hospital.

Circulation (with IV access and fluids):
Heart rate. Blood pressure. Hypovolaemia uncommon in initial stages of burn injury (if present, suspect delayed presentation, occult injury or cardiac disease). Peripheral temperature. Capillary refill. IV access preferably through unburnt skin (interosseous route may be required in children). Blood tests: FBC, U&Es, glucose, clotting screen, G&S. ECG/cardiac enzymes in high-tension electrical burns. ECG abnormalities more common if history of collapse/cardiac arrest associated with the injury. These patients require cardiac monitoring for 24 h.

Disability:
GCS/AVPU/ Pupillary reaction. If compromised, consider hypoxia, hypovolaemia or other injury (including head injury).

Exposure (with environment control):
Examine entire patient to estimate the percentage of total body surface area (TBSA) of the burn and check for concomitant injury. Prevent unnecessary/prolonged exposure, which can lead to hypothermia and burn depth extension.

Methods of percentage TBSA estimation:

1. Lund and Browder charts
    The younger the child, the greater the surface area of the head in proportion to the body. Use the relevant paediatric charts as necessary.
2. Rule of Nines
    Head 9%, arm 2 × 9%, torso 2 × 18% front and back, leg 2 × 18%, perineum 1%.
3. Palm of the (patient's) hand = 1%
    More useful for small or irregular burns.

Assessment of burn depth:

Superficial	+/– Blisters. Underlying tissue sensate (painful!) with bright red appearance. Blanching on digital pressure (painful procedure). Think sunburn!
Deeper partial thickness	Overlying epidermis and superficial dermis lost. Cherry red appearance of underlying dermis with punctate lesions. Fixed capillary staining on digital pressure with deeper dermal burns. Painful!
Full thickness	Eschar (thick/white +/– charring of surrounding tissues (flame burn) or leathery in appearance). Insensate. No bleeding to pinprick. Circumferential burns may impair limb circulation or restrict chest wall excursion.
Electrical burns	Arborisation pattern on skin. May have significant deep muscle injury with relatively normal looking overlying skin. Rhabdomyolysis, myoglobinuria

Fluid Resuscitation

Major burns associated with massive fluid loss, firstly, through the burn wound itself and secondly, loss of circulating volume (associated systemic inflammatory response). Fluid requirements calculated according to the percentage TSBA of burn. The British Burns Association recommends the Parkland Formula to calculate the crystalloid fluid requirements during the first 48 hours.

Parkland Formula: Resuscitation volume = 4 ml × wt (kg) × %TBSA.

Half given in the first 8 hours and half in the next 16 h, followed by the total amount in the second 24-h period.

Maintenance Fluid
IV maintenance required for all children and those adults unable to take oral fluids. NB limited glucose stores in children therefore use dextrose. Children also at risk of cerebral oedema so careful monitoring essential.

Hourly infusion rate for children = 4 ml/kg (first 10 kg) + 2 ml/kg (next 10 kg) + 1 ml/kg (every kg over 20).

Clinical Evaluation
Hourly heart rate, blood pressure, temperature and urine output. Aim for urinary output of 0.5–1 ml/kg/h. Complicated burns (e.g., high-tension electrical burns or inhalational injury) require increased fluids (urine output 1–2 ml/kg/h). The calculated fluid is a guide only and may require adjustment.

Analgesia
IV analgesia (opiates) should be provided for all burns patients.

Secondary survey
During this detailed examination of the patient, any other concomitant injuries should be identified, investigated and treated as appropriate.

Surgical Management of Burns

Immediate
Tracheostomy: This may be necessary to secure the airway.
Escharotomy: Should be performed in controlled environment in theatre under general anaesthetic. Mid-axial incisions used,

carefully sited around joints and near superficial nerves (e.g., the ulnar nerve at the medial epicondyle). Significant blood loss can occur.

Fasciotomy: Bone has high resistance, therefore in high-tension electrical burns, electrical energy is converted to heat within myofascial compartments leading to myonecrosis. Fasciotomies are required to relieve the pressure in these compartments, limiting myonecrosis and therefore the risk of acute tubular necrosis.

Burn excision
Early excision (<72h)
Early excision of the entire burn wound thought to limit systemic inflammatory response and improve outcome. Significant blood loss can occur. When considering early excision, determine cardiovascular stability of the patient, operative risk and potential morbidity of the wound itself if it were not removed rapidly. For burn wounds <30% TBSA, usually sufficient donor sites. For larger excisions, skin substitutes should be applied to remaining wound until autologous skin available. As a guide, each procedure should be limited to 2–3 h operative time. NB: Safer to perform a number of moderate procedures rather than one massive one.

Delayed Excision
May be indicated where burn depth unclear. More common in children. If burn shows little/no healing at 2 weeks, then excision and grafting indicated (reduces risk of hypertrophic scars).

Techniques
Tangential excision
Shaving of burn wound until bleeding bed obtained. Advantage: allows excision of the burn while preserving viable deep dermis. Disadvantage: associated with increased blood loss. Limit excisions to 18–25% TBSA at a time.

Fascial excision
Excision down to the underlying fascia. Advantages: Quick procedure with less blood loss than tangential excision. Disadvantages: poor appearance compared to tangential excision.

Excision and direct closure
Only really indicated for small full thickness burns

Skin cover
Autologous

SSG	Skin is usually meshed 1:1.5 but higher ratios may be used for very large burns and limited donor sites. The cosmetic appearance is inferior but it aids wound closure
FTSG	May be appropriate in small deep dermal or full thickness burns, particularly on the face and hands. Superior functional and cosmetic result but limited by the size of the defect

Allogenic
Cadaveric (glycerol or cryopreserved)
May be of use as a temporising method of wound cover. Both types require preparation before use. Glycerol preserved skin must be repeatedly washed in normal saline. Cyropreserved is gently warmed (less popular as theoretical infection risk). Some of the dermal elements may become incorporated in the recipient.

Xenograft
Pig skin. Temporising skin cover until other methods available.

Skin substitutes
Biobrane, Integra
Synthetic bilaminar skin substitutes, containing dermal components, collagen and connective tissue elements (GAGs). Varying degrees of incorporation into host bed.

Cultured keratinocytes
Spray delivery or sheet graft. Usually applied in combination with widely meshed SSG or dermal substitute for deeper burns.

Dressings

Simple	Jelonet, liquid paraffin (facial burns)
Silver containing	Flammazine
	Flammacerium
	Aquacel Ag

The benefit of silver containing preparations is to promote a sterile environment. They may however make burn depth assessment difficult if this has not been done prior to application.

Outcome

Delayed healing (more than 3 weeks) associated with hypertrophic scars. Scar management should start as soon as wounds healed to reduce risk of problematic hypertrophic scars and scar contracture. Includes scar massage, rehydration, pressure therapy and splints. Custom-made masks available for facial burns. These interventions continue until scar maturation has occurred (18–24/12). Follow up of patients in particular the paediatric populations who have not finished growth yet is vital.

Preservation of movement and function with vigorous exercise regimes aim to reduce morbidity associated with limited function.

Reduction in oedema with compression, movement, elevation and maximising lymphatic function.

Delayed surgical reconstruction aimed at resurfacing burned areas to improve cosmesis and function.

Chapter 8
Cleft Lip and Palate

Ivo Gwanmesia, Matthew Griffiths, and Jon Simmons

Cleft lip is a congenital abnormality of the primary palate involving the lip, alveolus and hard palate anterior to the incisive foramen. If the soft palate is involved, it is termed cleft lip and palate. It has an incidence of 1 in 750 live births.

Recognition

Usually seen as infants in the setting of a cleft lip and palate multidisciplinary team (Fig. 8.1).

History

When was the cleft diagnosed?
Where there any problems with the pregnancy?
Does the child have any feeding or breathing difficulties?
Are there any other congenital anomalies present?
Is there a family history of clefts?

I. Gwanmesia (✉)
Department of Plastic and Reconstructive Surgery,
Pan-Thames Training Scheme,
London, UK

S. Hettiaratchy et al. (eds.), *Plastic Surgery*,
DOI 10.1007/978-1-84882-116-3_8,
© Springer-Verlag London Limited 2012

57

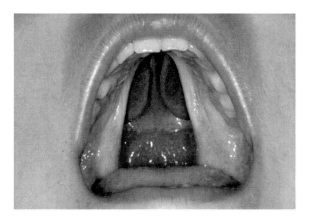

FIGURE 8.1 Complete cleft palate

AIM: by the end of history you should

1. Know about the general health of the child and any specific issues with breathing or feeding
2. Understand the extent of the cleft and structures involved
3. Identify any social/family factors that will require attention
4. Assess the parents understanding about the condition

Examination

Specific
Type of cleft: unilateral or bilateral, complete or incomplete,
primary or secondary, microform or forme fruste

Is the secondary palate involved?
Is the nose distorted?
Are the alveolar arches widely displaced? (The child may
require pre-surgical orthopaedics)

General

General body habitus
Normal weight for age – red book for height and weight
charts

Exclude presence of other congenital anomalies (their presence may be an indication of a syndromic cleft)

AIM: by the end of exam you should have

1. Assessed and documented the type of cleft and its extent
2. Identified any other anomalies
3. Assessed the child to determine suitability for surgery
4. Formulated a treatment strategy and timeline for treatment
5. Identified factors which may require treatment or investigation before surgery

Investigations

FBC, U&Es, group and save. Feeding assessment. Hearing assessment.

Treatment

Best carried out within a multidisciplinary team. Treatment requires surgical and non-surgical skills.

Non-surgical

Geneticist – screens for the presence of genetic conditions within the affected family
Clinical nurse specialist – advises parents on any feeding or breathing difficulties
Psychologist – to prepare older patient and family for treatment
Audiologist – assesses child's hearing

Surgical
An MDT involving – Plastic Surgeon, Maxillofacial Surgeon, ENT Surgeon, Orthodontist
Cleft lip repair is commonly performed at 3 months of age (or according to the rule of 10s; 10 kg, 10 g/dL of haemoglobin, 10 weeks of age) when the anaesthetic risk is much reduced. Primary rhinoplasty is also carried out at this time.

Cleft lip repair methods

Millard rotation advancement method
Tennison-Randall method

Cleft palate repair methods
Cleft palate is usually repaired at 6 months. The patient is also assessed for the need for grommets at this time. Other protocols exist (Fig. 8.2).

Direct closure for narrow clefts
Von Langenbeck technique (Fig. 8.3)
Furlow's double opposing Z-plasty

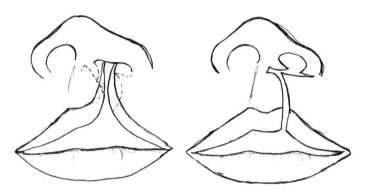

FIGURE 8.2 Millard technique for cleft lip repair

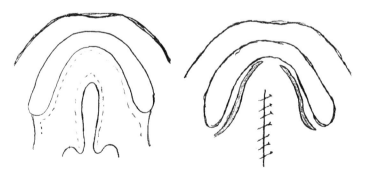

FIGURE 8.3 Von Langenbeck technique for palate repair

Veau-Wardill-Kilner technique
Intravelar veloplasty
Vomerine flaps

Complications of Repair

Infection
Dehiscence
Bleeding
Scarring
Whistle deformity of the lip
Breathing difficulties
Fistula formation of the palate
Velopharyngeal incompetence
Midfacial growth disturbance

Other Aspects of Cleft Lip and Palate Repair

Cleft lip and palate care varies from unit to unit, but the main points for patient management following cleft lip and palate repair include the following:

Speech and language assessment at 4–5 years
Alveolar bone grafting at 9–10 years (during the period of mixed dentition)
Orthodontic assessment and surgery at 11–18 years
Secondary rhinoplasty at skeletal maturity (may also be performed during growth)

Secondary Rhinoplasty

Cleft lip and palate patients usually still have residual deformities of the midfacial area after primary rhinoplasty. Treatment is carried out for functional and aesthetic reasons. Treatment is best carried out once all orthodontic treatment is completed. The patients would usually be between 16 and 19 years of age.

Some of the factors leading to these deformities include:

Intrinsic nasal factors

Deformed and depressed lower lateral cartilage
Deviated septum
Asymmetric nasal tip
Deviated columella
Asymmetric nasal bones and nasal pyramid

Extrinsic skeletal factors

Maxillary hypoplasia
Maxillary cleft (if not already corrected)
Lack of bony support for nasal base

A comprehensive and systematic assessment of the cleft deformity is necessary prior to initiating secondary rhinoplasty. This comprises of carrying out an *external* and *internal examination* of the nose.

External examination
Skeletal base support

Nasal base position (exclude retroposition)
Nasal base size and asymmetry
Columella length, shape and position
Size and shape of nostrils

Nasal dorsum

The degree of dorsal projection
Degree of asymmetry of the nasal pyramid
Degree of deviation of the nasal pyramid
The nasal width and length

Nasal tip and ala

Asymmetry in tip projection
Flattening of the ala on the affected side

Skin envelope
Position of any scars

Internal examination
The degree of septal cartilage deviation

Position of the footplates of the lower lateral cartilages
The size of the inferior turbinates
Is the caudal septum attached to the anterior nasal spine?
Are there any scars within the nasal vestibule?

Procedures carried out during secondary rhinoplasty include the following:
Bone grafting of maxillary defects, nasal bone osteotomies, submucous cartilaginous resection or septoplasty, the use of various cartilage grafts to provide support for the columella and to augment lower lateral cartilages, or as spreader grafts to correct a collapsed internal valve, various suture techniques to modify the position of the cartilages and skin flaps to lengthen the columella.

Outcomes

Utilising proven techniques in the context of the multi-disciplinary team, excellent cosmetic outcomes can and should be achieved. Speech quality as influenced by palatal development following repair requires treatment by speech and language therapists to maximise the potential for clear speech.

Velopharyngeal Dysfunction

The velopharynx is a rectangular structure that acts as a valve to separate the nasal and oral cavities during speech and swallowing.

- Causes of velopharyngeal dysfunction are classified as structural or neurologic impairment, and mechanical interference. It is seen in about 20% of cleft patients after palatoplasty.
- Structural impairment can result from submucous cleft palate, unrepaired cleft palate, short palate after palate repair, palatal fistula and tissue deficiency.
- Neurologic impairment can be due to neurologic disorders that impair the function of the muscular sphincter.

- Mechanical interference can result from large adenoids and tonsils.

Evaluation and Diagnosis

- Complete evaluation of velopharyngeal dysfunction includes assessment of perceptual speech, anatomy and physiology of the velopharyngeal complex.
- Assessment of perceptual speech is done by looking for hypernasality, nasal emission and compensatory articulation.
- Assessment of the anatomy of the velopharynx is through the use of nasendoscopy and videofluoroscopy.
- Assessment of the physiology of the velopharyngeal complex is performed by using nasometry.

Treatment

Treatment can be non-operative or operative.

- Non-operative treatment consists of speech therapy alone.
- Operative treatment includes pharyngeal flaps, pharyngoplasty, posterior pharyngeal wall augmentation, palate re-repair and velar muscle reconstruction (either through intravelar veloplasty or Furlow palatoplasty).

Complications of Surgical Correction of Velopharyngeal Dysfunction

These include postoperative bleeding, airway obstruction, obstructive sleep apnoea and possibly restriction of facial growth.

Chapter 9
Congenital Hand

Shehan Hettiaratchy and Jon Simmons

There is nothing a child with a congenital hand difference should not be allowed to do. Their difference is normal to them.

Recognition

Child with craniofacial syndrome with associated hand anomaly – try and identify the syndrome to determine the likely hand anomaly
Normal child with isolated limb difference
Normal child with multiple limb differences (Fig. 9.1)

History

Paediatric intro

Age, handedness if known
Pregnancy + delivery history
Growth and development
Associated medical problems and plan
Siblings/family history

S. Hettiaratchy (✉)
Department of Plastic and Reconstructive Surgery,
Imperial College Healthcare NHS Trust,
London, UK

S. Hettiaratchy et al. (eds.), *Plastic Surgery*,
DOI 10.1007/978-1-84882-116-3_9,
© Springer-Verlag London Limited 2012

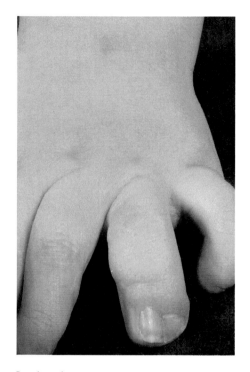

FIGURE 9.1 Syndactyly

Specific – Tailor this to what is age appropriate

When first noticed
Progression/worsening
Current state of hand function
Specific tasks unable to do
School performance
ADLs
Parents and child's goals

Risk factors

Teratogens
Twins
Large baby
Oligohydramnios
Family history

AIM: by the end of history you should have an idea of

1. The impact of the hand difference on the child
2. What has been done/achieved so far
3. Child's/parents' goals

Examination

Look

- Craniofacial syndrome:
- Apert's: complex syndactyly-varying degrees
- Crouzon's
- Carpenter's
- Pfeiffer's: broad toes/thumbs

One or multiple limbs:

- Symmetrical cleft hands/feet – typical cleft
- Different levels with absence – Constriction Ring Syndrome

Posture:

- Normal components abnormal posture – CP, BPI

Upper Limb normal posture:

- All components present
  - Hypoplastic: Poland's syndrome – check NAC/pectoralis major: Symbrachydactyly
  - Hyperplastic: hemihypertrophy
- Part missing
  - Hand present – intercalated
  - Hand absent – no nubbins – transverse arrest
  - Hand absent – nubbins – symbrachydactyly
- Hand present
  - Deviated at wrist/forearm short-longitudinal deficiency, check thumb as indicator if radial or ulnar
- Palm present
  - Cleft in palm – cleft hand

- Fingers present
  - All short – symbrachydactyly
  - Some short – brachydactyly
  - Radially deviated – little finger – clinodactyly
  - PIPJ flexion – camptodactyly
  - Fused – syndactyly
  - Abnormal position – arthrogryposis
  - Stiff – symphalangism
  - Hyperplastic – macrodactyly
  - Increase in number – radial/ulnar polydactyly – mirror hand
  - Decrease in number – symbrachydactyly
- Thumb
  - Small/absent – hypoplasia (Blauth)
  - Flexed – clasped thumb – trigger thumb

Feel/move

Check specific joint ranges and stability as indicated
Need to think about:

- Joint stability/stiffness – from shoulder downwards
- Length discrepancies – flex elbow to see if arm is short above or below/compare
- Correctability of any deviations – will influence the type of procedure/success
- Functional task
  - Holding pen/writing
  - Grasping cup (wide grip)
  - Handling toys

AIM: by the end of exam you should have an idea of

1. Specific functional limitations
2. Options, if any, for addressing them
3. Timing of any intervention given the age of the child

Investigations

Plain X-ray – after 6 months

Treatment

Principles

- Improve/preserve overall hand function, not individual joint movements.
- Cosmesis should not be achieved at the expense of function.
- For the child the hand is normal, how they adapt may exceed what is expected.
- Timing is critical as an intervention too early may lead to recurrence. Too late may not fully correct the problem.

What to treat

- To release abnormally joined structures (e.g., syndactyly)
- To join abnormally separated structures (e.g., cleft hand)
- To correct deviation (longitudinal deficiencies)
- To prevent future deviation (clinodactyly)
- To reconstruct a missing part
- To remove an extra/duplicated part

Options for treatment
Non-surgical
Physiotherapy

- May help stiffness/contractures/instability
- Splintage may be a useful adjunct for certain conditions (longitudinal deficiencies)

Botox
May have a role in arthrogryposis to balance agonist/antagonist

Surgical general timing
Techniques will depend on the condition being treated and the intended aim. Timing:

<1 year: syndactyly where growth might be affected
>1 year: other syndactyly
>2 years: microvascular surgery
2–4 years: clinodactyly – physiolysis)

Specific procedures
Syndactyly release
Stage if both sides of a digit are involved

Various techniques – mainly interdigitating triangular flaps for digits and some form of dorsal flap for commisure. Buck-Gramcko paronychial flaps. Some form of skin grafting often needed – tend to be FTSG.

First web release
Seen in association with clasped thumb/hypoplasia. Is it skin or adductor? Splintage first.
If very tight may need surgery

- Skin – 4 flap z-plasty
- Adductor – release

Clinodactyly
Operate if >45°/progressing. Options:

- Physiolysis – if still growing (best done 2–4 years) then rely on the finger growing straight and correcting
- Osteotomy – if no longer growing/physiolysis has not worked

Trigger thumb

Often not diagnosed early (neonates clasp their thumb).
Palpate nodule in FPL (Notta's node). May get stuck in flexion or extension.
May resolve before 2 years old. Otherwise operate; release radial part of A1 to avoid injury to the oblique pulley.

Clasped thumb

Splintage/therapy
If skin short may need transposition flap from radial border of index finger
EPL reconstruction

Thumb hypoplasia

Critical is quality of CMCJ and stability.
If stable, then aim is to reconstruct around the CMCJ (i.e., improve adductor function).
If unstable/missing may be better to pollicise.

Thumb duplication

Choose which is the better formed duplicate and use that as basis for reconstruction. May need to reconstruct IPJ/MPJ stability, FPL, EPL and delineate digital nerves (may need interneural dissection).

Radial longitudinal deficiency

Targets for treatment are to improve wrist/hand position and thumb reconstruction while maximising ulna growth. This can often be conflicting – options to place the carpus on the end of the radius may damage the ulnar physis and compromise growth.

Options:

- Centralisation
- Radialisation (Buck-Gramcko)
- Vascularised physis transfer (Vilkki) – 2nd MT taken as a free flap
- Manipulation only (Ezaki)

Risks and Complications

These will depend on the surgery and timing. Recurrence of the problem is often an issue in certain conditions.

Aetiology

Upper limb and hand development between the 4th and 12th week of gestation initiated by fibroblast growth factors. Development occurs along three axes. Proximal to distal (Apical ectodermal ridge), anterior to posterior (zone of pola- rising activity) and dorsal to ventral (wingless gene encoded protein). Apoptosis is responsible for separating the digits.

Classifications

IFSSH Swanson classification
Blauth thumb hypoplasia Syndactyly
Bayne-Radial/Ulnar dysplasia

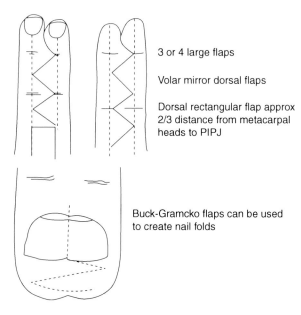

3 or 4 large flaps

Volar mirror dorsal flaps

Dorsal rectangular flap approx
2/3 distance from metacarpal
heads to PIPJ

Buck-Gramcko flaps can be used
to create nail folds

FIGURE 9.2 Syndactyly flap design. The commisural flap has many
variations

Controversies

Timing of treatment
Commisure flap design in syndactyly
FTSG vs. SSG vs. open finger technique in syndactyly (Fig. 9.2).

Chapter 10
Craniosynostosis

Ivo Gwanmesia and Matthew Griffiths

Craniosynostosis is the premature fusion of one or more cranial sutures. It is classified according to the suture(s) involved. It can be either syndromic or deformational. It has an incidence of 1 in 2,000 live births.

Recognition

A child with an abnormal skull and face presenting to a craniofacial multidisciplinary team (Fig. 10.1).

History

- When was the deformity initially noticed?
- Where there any problems with the pregnancy?
- Has there been an improvement in the shape of the head over time?
- Is there a positive family history of abnormal head shapes?
- Is the child developing normally?
- Have there been any signs of raised intracranial pressure? (Irritability, vomiting, tense fontanelles, seizures, papilloedema)

I. Gwanmesia (✉)
Department of Plastic and Reconstructive Surgery,
Pan-Thames Training Scheme,
London, UK

S. Hettiaratchy et al. (eds.), *Plastic Surgery*,
DOI 10.1007/978-1-84882-116-3_10,
© Springer-Verlag London Limited 2012

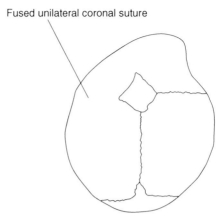

Fused unilateral coronal suture

FIGURE 10.1 Plagiocephaly – fused coronal suture

Examination

Specific
Look

- What is the shape of the skull?
- Are the ears in a similar position?
- Are the orbits symmetrical? – Patients with unilateral coronal synostosis typically have a wind-swept unilateral orbit due to the anterior position of the sphenoid
- Is there any evidence of papilloedema?
- Are the cheeks symmetrical?
- Is the nose deviated?
- Is the chin in the midline?

Feel

- Is the anterior fontanelle open?
- Is the posterior fontanelle open?
- Is there a palpable ridge?
- Do the sternocleidomastoid muscles feel normal and is there a full range of neck movement?

General

- Are they any abnormalities of the limbs?
- Are there any cardiac abnormalities?

Investigations

- Plain X-ray – sufficient to identify the affected suture(s); the beaten-copper appearance is an indication of raised intracranial pressure.
- CT scan – gold standard for imaging, however comes with a higher dose of radiation. Useful for detecting the presence of Arnold-Chiari malformations seen in Crouzon syndrome.

Treatment

Always within the context of a multidisciplinary team.

Non-surgical

- Geneticist: Determines evidence of a potential syndromic or a familial pattern of inheritance
- Neuropsychologist: determines patient's underlying brain function which serves as a benchmark for any postoperative changes
- Paediatrician: assesses patient's general well-being
- Paediatric ophthalmologist: excludes the presence of papilloedema

Positioning and the use of orthotic devices are useful for positional plagiocephaly.

Surgical

Indications for surgery include significant cranial and facial asymmetry, elevated intracranial pressure (ICP) and neuropsychologic disorders.

In most cases of single suture craniosynostosis, the indication for surgery is the degree of cranial and/or facial asymmetry.

Trigonocephaly

Premature fusion of the metopic suture.

Has an incidence of 1 in 10,000 live births and account for 10–20% of all cases of single suture synotoses.

Affected patients usually present with a keel-shaped forehead with a palpable ridge and hypotelorism.

Surgical correction involves the elevation of a bifrontal flap, excision of the synostoses, calvarial remodelling through the use of kerfs with radial osteotomies and the use of bone grafts if the defect is greater than 2 cm. Some units may in addition use orthotic devices to assist with calvarial remodelling.

Scaphocephaly

Most common form of unilateral craniosynostosis. It is the premature fusion of the sagittal suture.

Has an incidence of 1 in 2,000 live births.

Patients present with a long head.

Surgical correction usually involves the elevation of frontal, parietal and occipital bone flaps and remodelling of the flaps by osteotomies.

Some units use orthotic devices to assist in achieving the desired head shape.

Plagiocephaly

It is the premature fusion of a unilateral coronal suture.

It has an incidence of 1 in 4,500.

The features include a retropositioned forehead on the affected side, a raised superior orbital ridge, a laterally positioned lateral canthus, a nasal root deviated towards the affected orbit, a prominent cheek on the affected side and the chin deviated away from the affected orbit.

Surgical treatment involves the elevation of a bifrontal bone flap and three-quarter orbital osteotomies. The orbits are advanced unequally to correct the orbital deformity. Bone grafts may or may not be used.

Brachycephaly

Premature fusion of the coronal sutures.

It has an incidence of 1 in 2,500 live births and accounts for 25% of single suture synostosis.

Patients present with a long head, flattening of the occiput, skull widening and some have been described as tower head 'turribrachycephaly'.

Surgical correction involves elevation of frontal and occipital bone flaps and correction with radial osteotomies.

Lambdoidal plagiocephaly
Premature fusion of a single lambdoid suture.
It is the least common of all the single suture synostosis, accounting for less than 5% of all synostosis.
Patients present with a flattened occiput on the affected side, the ear on the affected side is posterior compared to the contralateral ear, and there is bossing of the forehead on the affected side.
Surgical correction involves the raising of an occipital bone flap and radial osteotomies with or without the use of springs to correct the head shape.

Surgical complications of calvarial remodelling
Complications are acute and delayed.
Acute complications include blood loss, dural tear with CSF leak, infection and respiratory infections. Delayed complications are predominantly those of relapse and scalp scarring.

Syndromic Craniosynostosis

Apert syndrome (acrocephalosyndactyly type I)
Autosomal dominant inheritance
Incidence of 1 in 25,000 to 1 in 100,000
Typically present with bilateral coronal synostosis, with turribrachycephaly skull deformity, midface hypoplasia and complex syndactyly

Crouzon syndrome (acrocephalosyndactyly type II)
Autosomal dominant inheritance
Incidence of 1 in 10,000 to 1 in 25,000
Typically present with bilateral coronal synostosis with severe midface hypoplasia, exorbitism
There is no syndactyly

Saetre-Chotzen syndrome (acrocephalosyndactyly III)
Autosomal dominant inheritance
Incidence of 1 in 10,000

Features include unilateral coronal synostosis, low-set hair-line, ear abnormalities and incomplete simple syndactyly of the hands

Carpentar syndrome (acrocephalosyndactyly type IV)
Autosomal recessive inheritance
Incidence of 1 in 10,000
Features include sagittal or bicoronal synostosis, widely spaced eyes, hydrocephalus, some have heart defects.

Pfeiffer syndrome (acrocephalosyndactyly V)
Autosomal dominant inheritance
Incidence of 1 in 15,000
Features include coronal synostosis, midface hypoplasia and limb abnormalities including broad thumbs and toes (Fig.10.2).

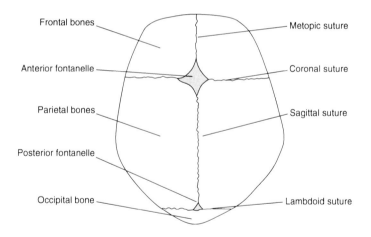

FIGURE 10.2 Sutures and bones of the normal skull

Chapter 11
Dupuytren's Disease

Shehan Hettiaratchy and Jon Simmons

Benign fibroproliferative disease of unknown aetiology. Important to identify the patient with a diathesis/aggressive disease. The patient must realise that no interventions can cure, they only buy a variable disease-free interval.

Recognition

Male patient over 50 with ulnar sided contracture of fingers. Often bilateral, be aware of early onset, recurrent and extra-palmar disease (Fig. 11.1).

Differentials include: ulnar nerve lesion, joint contracture, scar contracture.

History

Hand intro – Age, occupation, handedness, hobbies, musical instruments and interference with these.

S. Hettiaratchy (✉)
Department of Plastic and Reconstructive Surgery,
Imperial College Healthcare NHS Trust,
London, UK

S. Hettiaratchy et al. (eds.), *Plastic Surgery*,
DOI 10.1007/978-1-84882-116-3_11,
© Springer-Verlag London Limited 2012

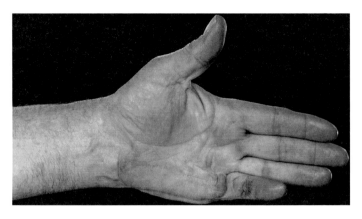

FIGURE 11.1 Dupuytrens disease

Disease specific

1. Specific problems the patients has, what cannot they do, what do they want to achieve?
2. How long have they had it? Progression? Why are they seeking treatment now?
3. Any pain/numbness/tingling?
4. Any previous treatment/surgery? When and what?
5. Any other sites affected? (extra palmar, feet-Lederhosen, penis – Peyronie's).

Risk factors

1. Family history – who, at what age, progression/treatment
2. Smoking – how much and for how long
3. EtOH – how much? How long?
4. IDDM
5. Epilepsy – what medications?
6. Diathesis – aggressive/young/FHx/ectopic

General – Previous medical history/drug history, especially any anti-coagulants, aspirin, etc. social history including home circumstances, support mechanisms

AIM: by the end of history you should have

1. Determined how aggressive the disease is (influences type of surgery and outcome).
2. Assessed what the patient's main complaint is and what they want to do about it.
3. Assessed the practicality of surgery for the patient, and suitability for surgery.

Examination

General – Sit across table, expose patients arms below the elbow. Examine both hands together.
Look

- *Palmar surface* – Digits affected, previous scars (including forearm), skin pits, obvious nodules
- *Dorsal surface* – Garrod's pads any guttering or wasting of first dorsal interosseous (ulnar nerve lesion)
- *Table top test* – Quick gross assessment of disease/amount of MPJ/PIPJ contracture. Patients places hands as flat as possible on the table, palms down.

Feel/move
Overview
One hand at a time. Palpate all cords under tension as it makes them more obvious. Hyperextend fingers and look for obvious cords. Quickly palpate palm, affected fingers, thumb, first web space. Check first web and hand span (compare both sides – limited span suggests involvement of the natatory bands). Check palm for nodules.

Disease extent/configuration
Examine each affected digit in detail. Determine if it is only palmar disease or disease in the finger. Identify affected cords. Identify a spiral cord as it increases the risk of digital nerve injury (displaces NVB).

Range of movement using Goniometer
Check ROM. Measure MPJ extension. Flex MPJ (eliminates effect of short intrinsics) and measure PIPJ ROM. Note active and passive range. Note attenuation of the central slip (i.e., is passive extension of PIPJ greater than active extension). Attenuation increases the risk of joint contracture.

- Assess the skin in the affected digits – will a graft be required?
- Check and comment on sensation

AIM: by the end of exam you should consider

1. Extent of disease
2. Type of surgery required (soft tissue/joints)
3. Whether FTSG will be required
4. If there is a spiral cord – potential risk to the nerves

Investigations

Only as indicated on the basis of clinical findings and history. Blood work on the basis of co-morbidities. Nerve conduction studies if considering peripheral nerve lesion.

Treatment

Options

1. Watch and wait
2. Non-surgical
3. Surgical

When to treat

1. PIPJ contracture – greater than 30° (McFarlane)
2. MPJ – no absolute figure, consider individual patient and disease progression
3. Significant interference with activities
4. Aggressive disease

Non-surgical treatment

1. Splintage – no evidence of effect
2. Steroids (nodules) – not universally accepted
3. Collagenases – ?future. FDA approved for treatment. Role and RCT awaited.

Surgical

1. Fasciotomy
   Simple division of the cord; done under LA; best for palmar disease
   Advantages: quick, simple, effective
   Disadvantages: high recurrence rate; risk of DN injury in finger/thumb
   Complications: DN injury; incomplete release
   Indication: elderly patient, pre-tendinous cord, unfit for surgery
2. Limited fasciectomy
   Removal of affected tissue, leaving behind unaffected fascia
   Advantage: lower recurrence rate than fasciotomy
   Disadvantages: needs GA/regional block; higher recurrence than dermofasciectomy
   Complications: wound problems, DN injury, recurrence
   Indication: most primary, non-rapidly progressing disease
3. Dermofasciectomy
   Removal of affected skin and underlying cords
   Adv: lowest (if any) recurrence
   Disadv: donor site/FTSG take
   Complications: graft failure; donor site problems
   Indications: recurrent disease; aggressive disease in the young; extensive skin involvement

PIPJ management
Aggressive surgical release may cause more scarring and limit movement.

Release check rein ligaments and accessory collateral ligaments in combination with gentle passive manipulation. Approximately half the correction is usually lost over the first 6 months. Recurrence is more likely if central slip attenuated; correcting attenuation offers limited benefit.

Skin incisions

Bruner

Adv: start dissection in normal tissue, Y-V allows extra skin to be imported

Disadv: tips of flap vulnerable, limited skin imported, does not re-orientate dermal fascia

Skoog

Adv: multiple z-plasties importing skin, z-plasties realign dermal fascia

Disadv: harder to reopen, dissection started in abnormal tissue

Palm is often left open (McCash technique)

Post-operative management

Fasciotomy	Minimal dressing; nightsplint 6/12
Limited fasciectomy	Palmar: nightsplint 6/12, Finger: splint day and night 6/52 then night to 6/12
Dermofasciectomy	Splint day and night 6/52 then night to 6/12

Risks/Complications

1–3% nerve injury depending on procedure
5% delayed healing
<1% ischaemia

Outcome

Fasciotomy – 100% by ??
Fasciectomy – 45% by 5 years
Dermofasciectomy – 0–35% by 5 years

History

First described by Astley Cooper in 1777. First released by Baron Guillaume Dupuytren in 1831. Hueston described diathesis in 1961.

Anatomy

Dupuytren's disease involves the normal fascial structures of the palm and digits (Fig. 11.2)

Pre-tendinous band: Pre-tendinous cord

Natatory ligament: Natatory cord

Superficial volar fascia: Central cord

Lateral digital sheet: Lateral cord

Spiral cord is formed from proximal to distal by the pre-tendinous band; oblique or spiral band; the lateral digital sheet; Grayson's ligament.

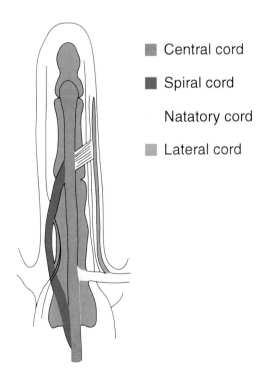

■ Central cord

■ Spiral cord

  Natatory cord

■ Lateral cord

FIGURE 11.2 Dupuytrens cords

Pathophysiology

Luck described 3 phases; proliferative/involutional/residual

Proliferative
Random accumulation of fibroblasts in a whorl like pattern – nodules

Involutional
Differentiating fibroblasts in the presence of tension causes aggregation of fibroblasts along these tension lines causing cords. Myofibroblast differentiation.

Residual
Cords become relatively acellular.

Key Evidence

Hueston, J.T. Limited fasciectomy for Dupuytren's contracture. Plast. Reconstr. Surg. 27:569, 1961.

McCash, R.The open palm technique in Dupuytren's contracture. Br. J. Plast. Surg. 17:271, 1964.

McFarlane, R.M. Clinical perspective on the origin and spread of Dupuytren's disease. J. Hand Surg. (Am.) 27:385, 2002.

Swartz, William M. M.D.; MOC-PS(SM) CME Article: Dupuytren's Disease; Plastic and Reconstructive Surgery; Volume 121(4) Supplement, April 2008, pp 1–10.

Chapter 12
Facial Palsy

Ivo Gwanmesia, Farida Ali, and Jon Simmons

Facial palsy is the paralysis of the seventh (facial) cranial nerve. It can be unilateral or bilateral. There are multiple causes.

Recognition

Patient (adult or infant) presenting with facial weakness and asymmetry (Fig. 12.1).

History

- When was the weakness/deformity initially noticed?
- Are there any known causes?
- Is there a history of associated trauma?
- Has the patient had any previous treatment?
- What problems is the patient having?

I. Gwanmesia (✉)
Department of Plastic and Reconstructive Surgery,
Pan-Thames Training Scheme,
London, UK

S. Hettiaratchy et al. (eds.), *Plastic Surgery*,
DOI 10.1007/978-1-84882-116-3_12,
© Springer-Verlag London Limited 2012

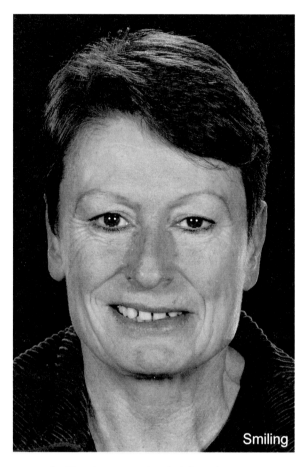

Smiling

FIGURE 12.1 Smiling demonstrating facial weakness

- Is there eye pain?
- Does the patient experience any difficulties with hearing?
- Does the patient experience any difficulties with speech and feeding?

Examination

(Top to bottom examination of the face)

Specific
Look

- Hairline and position
- Forehead wrinkles
- Brow position
- Presence of nasal deviation with evidence of external valve collapse
- Malar flattening and ptosis
- Increase in length of upper lip
- Asymmetry of the mouth

Feel

- Sensation along the ophthalmic, maxillary and mandibular branches of the trigeminal nerve
- Palpate the temporalis muscle, asking the patient to bite hard at the same time

Move

- Ask patient to elevate forehead and brows
- Ask patient to close eyes
- Ask patient to blow out cheeks
- Check for Cottle's sign (in order to exclude internal valve collapse)
- Ask patient to show his/her teeth
- Ask patient to contract the neck muscles

General
Complete general physical examination.

Investigations

Investigations are usually directed towards cause (if known). They are broadly classified as etiologic, prognostic and topographic.

Aetiologic
Blood tests

- Serologic studies for: syphilis, diabetes, hyper- and hypothyroidism
- Viral titres for: herpes, varicella zoster and Epstein Barr virus

Imaging

- X-rays of the mastoid
- CT scan to detect intracranial, intratemporal and extratemporal tumours of the facial nerve
- MRI scan with Gadolinium will delineate the course of the facial nerve

Prognostic
Used to determine if facial nerve regeneration has begun

Nerve Excitability Test – Performed with nerve stimulator. A 3ma difference between the two sides of the face is regarded as an abnormal result.

Maximal Stimulation Test – Also performed with nerve stimulator. Abnormal test result is any difference in facial movement between the two sides of the face.

Electroneurography – Current is delivered to the stylomastoid foramen, sufficient to evoke maximum response of the facial muscles. A difference of 95% in the evoked compound muscle action potential between the two sides of the face is sufficient to indicate unsatisfactory return of facial function following regeneration.

Electromyography – Should only be considered after 3 weeks if no recovery is clinically apparent. Useful in detecting early return of facial nerve function.

Topographic – CT and MRI scans: useful for locating the site of a lesion.

Treatment

Treatment is broadly classified into watchful waiting, medical and surgical

Watchful waiting
Indicated for mild cases of facial palsy. Eighty percent of patients treated this way begin to recover within 3 weeks

Medical treatment
Corticosteroids – remains controversial but patients usually recover facial movement to a House-Brackmann Grade 1 or 2

Surgical treatment

Direct Nerve Repair/transposition
Primary nerve repair (intracranial, intratemporal, extratemporal)
Interpositional nerve graft (most commonly sural nerve)
Cross face nerve graft (sural nerve)
Hypoglossal facial nerve transfer
Hypoglossal facial nerve jump graft (sural nerve)

Free Muscle Transfer (with cross-face nerve graft)
Free muscle flap (gracilis, latissimus dorsi, pectoralis minor, serratus anterior) with cross-face sural nerve graft

Regional Muscle Transposition
Temporalis muscle transposition
Masseter muscle transposition
Digastric muscle transposition

Static Facial Support
Browlift
Blepharoplasty
Upper lid gold weight
Lower lid repositioning and support
Lip and cheek support (fascia lata, Goretex)

Chapter 13
Maxillofacial Trauma

Farida Ali, Ivo Gwanmesia, and Jon Simmons

All cases should be managed as per ATLS guidelines. The principles of management in facial fractures are accurate diagnosis on clinical examination and radiography, followed by early surgical treatment. It is no longer common practice to wait for the swelling to settle before surgical treatment.

Recognition

Maxillofacial trauma may involve bony injury, soft tissue injury or a combination. Though facial injuries themselves are not usually life threatening, three life-threatening emergencies may occur: respiratory obstruction, aspiration and haemorrhage. Ten percent of patients with facial fractures have an associated cervical spine injury and 10% have an associated ocular injury. Early CT scanning is essential in identifying the configuration of bony injury and planning surgical intervention (Fig. 13.1).

F. Ali (✉)
Department of Plastic and Reconstructive Surgery,
St George's Hospital,
London, UK

S. Hettiaratchy et al. (eds.), *Plastic Surgery*,
DOI 10.1007/978-1-84882-116-3_13,
© Springer-Verlag London Limited 2012

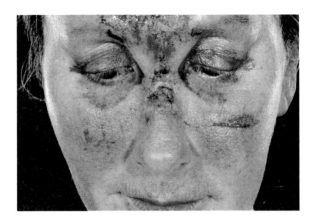

FIGURE 13.1 Facial injuries

History

General

- The exact mechanism of injury – high-energy vs. low energy, blunt or penetrating object, e.g., car, windscreen or sharp object
- Loss of consciousness
- Neck pain (cervical spine injury in 10%)
- Alcohol intake (may mask head injury)
- General health
- Allergies/medications
- Smoking history
- Last oral intake

Specific
Upper third

- Frontal sinus and anterior cranial fossa: Ask about pain, CSF rhinorrhoea
- Altered vision: Ask about loss of vision, blurred or double vision (orbital floor, zygomatic fractures)

Middle third

- Orbits: Remember, ocular injury is present in 10% of patients with facial fractures
- Zygoma: Swelling usually obvious
- Maxilla: Ask about dentition (missing/loose)
- Nose: Deformity/deviation (rule out a previous history of fracture)

Lower third

- Mandible: Dentition
- Trismus: do they have pain on movement of the mandible? Zygomatic arch fractures (impingement on coronoid process) or mandibular fractures involving the coronoid process
- Occlusion: Is occlusion normal? Ask them if their teeth meet normally anteriorly and posteriorly

Sensation

- Forehead numbness (supratrochlear and supraorbital nerves)
- Upper lip and teeth (infraorbital nerve)
- Lower lip and teeth (mental nerve)

Facial lacerations

Ask about abnormal facial movement. The position of the laceration will guide you to specific branches of the facial nerve. The parotid duct may also be injured in lacerations of the cheek.

Other injuries

This is particularly important with high-energy facial injuries. Consider chest, abdominal and long bone injuries, all of which may be a source of significant haemorrhage.

AIM: by the end of history you should have

1. Identified symptoms and correlated these with injuries
2. Understood the exact mechanism of injury and anticipated likely injuries
3. Systematically considered different levels of injury

Examination

Primary survey

You may be shown a photograph of a patient with major disruption of the face (e.g., gunshot, blast injury). Do not be distracted by gross facial injuries. Approach the scenarios as per ATLS guidelines!

Airway (with cervical spine control)
Airway obstruction: Blood, vomitus and/or foreign bodies (including teeth) can obstruct the airway and should be removed ASAP. Tongue may drop back if mandibular fracture associated with a flail segment.

A protected airway should be secured as soon as possible. Endo-tracheal intubation can be extremely difficult in patients with major maxillofacial injury. Nasotracheal intubation should be avoided in any patient that may have cribriform plate fractures.

Breathing (with 100% oxygen via non-rebreather bag)
Patients unable to maintain oxygenation require intubation and ventilation. Reduced conscious level, from intoxication or head injury, may also impair respiratory effort. Patients who have aspirated are at high risk and may well require ventilatory support. Failure of intubation requires cricothyroidotomy, which is a temporary measure until a definitive surgical airway can be secured.

Circulation (with IV access)
Obtain IV access with two large-bore cannulae and draw blood for analysis.

Control of life threatening haemorrhage may include:

Manual reduction of the fractures (temporary measure)
Packing of the nasal and oral cavities
Foley catheters to control bleeding from the nasopharyngeal region
Facial bandaging (not commonly used today)

Embolisation or ligation of the source arteries may be required. If embolisation is not available, transantral ligation of the internal maxillary arteries and ligation of the facial arteries may help control bleeding. Ligation of the external carotid artery has been used as a last resort.

Disability
GCS/AVPU/pupillary reaction.

Exposure
This should be a brief examination to rule out any concomitant injury.

Secondary survey
Once the patient has been stabilised and the primary survey completed, a detailed examination of the maxillofacial region should be performed. Be systematic: start at the top and work your way down.

Look

• Examine the patient from the front, from the top of the head (bird's eye view) and from below (worm's eye view).

Face

• Lacerations and soft tissue
• Facial swelling, asymmetry or deformity
• Facial elongation – midface fractures
• Loss of malar prominence – most easily identified from above – zygomatic arch fractures

Orbits

• Periorbital ecchymosis (bilateral or Panda eyes associated with BOS fracture)
• Enophthalmos – may be more noticeable from above
• Orbital dystopia – vertical height discrepancy of the globe – orbital blowout fracture (floor involved, rim spared)
• Subconjunctival haemorrhage (posterior margin visible? If not, consider anterior cranial fossa /orbital fractures)

Nose

- Nasal deformity
- Septal haematoma
- CSF rhinorrhoea (base of skull (BOS) fracture)

Ears

- Haematoma (needs drainage to prevent cauliflower ear deformity)
- Mastoid ecchymosis (Battle's sign) associated with BOS fracture. Usually occurs after days
- CSF otorrhoea (BOS fracture)

Intraoral

Do not forget to look inside the mouth for:

- Degree of mouth opening: limited with trismus. TMJ dislocation/fracture
- Teeth: missing, loose, malocclusion
- Haematoma of the palate (maxillary fractures) or upper buccal sulcus (zygomatic fractures)
- Intraoral lacerations
- Parotid duct injury (may see blood at Stenson's duct (opposite upper second molar)

Palpation

Start at the skull and work systematically, feeling for tenderness, steps, crepitus (sinus fractures) or abnormal movement at suture lines.

Le Fort fractures of the midface (may be asymmetrical) (Fig. 13.2).

I   – maxilla only – floating palate
II – pyramidal fracture
III – craniofacial disassociation

Neurological examination
Motor

Check each branch of the facial nerve

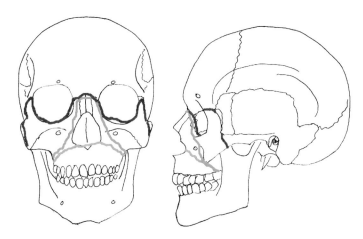

FIGURE 13.2 Le Fort classification

Sensory

Forehead (supratrochlear and supraorbital)
Cheek, upper lip and upper teeth (infraorbital)
Lower lip and lower teeth (mental)

Vision

Relative Afferent Pupillary Defect (RAPD).
Visual acuity, HESS chart
Snellen chart, finger counting, perception of light
Visual fields
Extra-ocular eye movements
Limitation of upward gaze associated with diplopia suggests entrapment of the inferior oblique muscle (orbital floor fractures)

Investigations

Once life-threatening injuries have been addressed and the patient has been stabilised, further investigations may be performed.

X-rays

Be guided by your clinical findings. There are many different views that have been used to image the facial skeleton. Waters: Oblique AP of orbital rims and maxilla. Panorex: mandible, OPG.

CT

Most units managing maxillofacial trauma now use CT scan (+/– 3D reconstruction) to accurately delineate complex facial fractures and aid treatment planning.

Treatment

Medical

Broad-spectrum antibiotic cover (fractures open to oral cavity, dog/human bites) and tetanus.

Surgical
Soft tissue injuries

Wound debridement (including scrubbing for road rash), minimal wound margin excision, copious lavage and layered repair should be performed.

Lacrimal duct

Should be performed by an experienced oculoplastic surgeon. Repair over a stent, (removed after minimum of 3/12).

Facial nerve injury

Nerve branches readily identifiable lateral to a vertical line from the outer canthus and should be repaired directly under magnification (loupe or microscope). Beyond this limit, there is no indication for surgical repair (nerve branches small and may have adequate crossover between except frontal and mandibular branches).

Parotid duct laceration

Options include repair over a stent (removed after 2-3/52), ligation or reimplantation into the buccal mucosa.

Maxillofacial fractures

Detailed management of specific fractures is outside the remit of this book. The following addresses the basic principles:

1. Accurate diagnosis through thorough clinical examination and radiographic evaluation
2. Early single stage surgery with
   (a) Adequate exposure of bony fragments
   (b) Rigid fixation and the immediate use of bone graft as necessary
   (c) Finally, re-suspension and reconstruction of the soft tissues

Adequate exposure

Take advantage of any pre-existing lacerations, which may be useful to approach fractures. However, additional incisions may be required to aid visualisation, reduction and/ or fixation of fractures.

Methods of fixation

Intermaxillary fixation

Requires tooth-bearing segments of maxilla and mandible on either side of the fracture fragments. May also act as a splint to maintain the relative position of the maxilla and mandible while a distant fracture heals.

Intraosseous wiring

Though not rigid, it may be of use at the ZF suture and infraorbital rim.

Plate fixation

Low profile monocortical plates now generally advocated for most fractures in the maxillofacial region.

Bone grafting

If >5 mm bone gap present, bone graft usually indicated. The orbital floor also frequently requires bone graft to reconstruct the bony orbit, reposition and support the globe. Donor sites: calvarium (outer table; thin membranous bone; good for orbital floor), rib, iliac crest.

Re-suspension and reconstruction of the soft tissues

Re-suspension of the soft tissues reduces facial oedema, prevents soft tissue contracture and therefore the risk of postoperative asymmetry. Reconstruction of soft tissue defects provides optimal environment for bone healing.

Condylar fractures of the mandible – treatment is controversial

Conservative: Undisplaced fractures. Soft diet

Intermaxillary fixation: Adequate dentition required

ORIF: Indicated with TMJ dislocation, significant displacement or bilateral fractures with anterior open bite

Chapter 14
Gynaecomastia

Robert Caulfield and Jon Simmons

Gynaecomastia is the abnormal breast development in the male, with increase in ductal tissue and stroma.

Recognition

Can present at any age: neonatal, pubertal or senile gynaeco-mastia (See history below). Recognised by excess of breast tissue +/− excess skin, usually predominately subareolar in location (Fig. 14.1).

History

General
Age, time of onset, duration, progression, occupation, inter-ference with lifestyle and occupation.

R. Caulfield (✉)
Specialist Registrar in Plastic and Reconstructive Surgery,
Pan-Thames Training Scheme,
London, UK

S. Hettiaratchy et al. (eds.), *Plastic Surgery*,
DOI 10.1007/978-1-84882-116-3_14,
© Springer-Verlag London Limited 2012

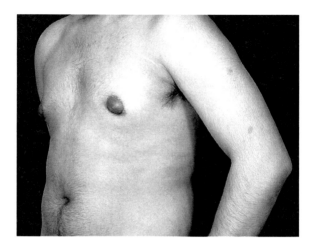

FIGURE 14.1 Gynaecomastia

Specific
These questions depend on age of patient (hence likely cause).

- Age of onset ? (N.B. If pubertal: 75% of pubertal males affected and 75% of these resolve within 2 years)
- Unilateral or bilateral?
- Area affected – central subareolar or diffuse breast enlargement?
- Excess tissue firm (glandular) or soft (adipose)?
- Any previous treatment /surgery?
- Patient's expectations about outcome vs. awareness of limitations of treatment and risks

Risk factors

- Smoking (marijuana)
- Medications (Spironolactone, Cimetidine, Digoxin, Metoclopramide, Tricyclics, Methyldopa, androgen blockers, e.g., Zoladex, Oestrogens)
- Alcohol consumption (Risk of cirrhosis – imbalance in oestrogen metabolism)
- Weight gain /obesity (Increased production of oestrogen in adipose tissue)

- Pre-existing renal disease (Causes increased LH and oestrogens)
- Pre-existing general disability (Interferes with pituitary-hypothalamic axis, e.g., burns)

General
Full medical and drug history

- Pituitary disorders (causes decreased GnRH, FH and LH)
- Symptoms/signs of thyroid disease (hyperthyroidism causes increased serum binding globulin and less free androgen – hence oestrogen/androgen imbalance)
- Male breast cancer (family history, specific breast lumps)
- Liver disease (cirrhosis)
- Renal disease (increased LH and oestrogens)
- Testes (seminomas, teratomas and choriocarcinomas cause increased hCG; Leydig, Sertoli and granulosa theca cell cause increased oestrogen)

AIM: by the end of history you should know

1. What the likely cause is: physiological, pathological or pharmaceutical
2. Need for additional investigations/treatment of any pathological causes
3. Treatment/progress to date
4. What the patient hopes to achieve
5. Chances of surgery meeting these objectives

Examination

Look
Evidence of general obesity. Any overt signs of hyperthyroidism, cirrhosis, renal disease, testicular masses

Thyroid
Examine for goitre – diffuse/localised enlargement

Breast
Examine both breasts and axillae

- Unilateral of bilateral
- Subareolar or diffuse enlargement (grade – see below)
- Specific breast lumps and any axillary nodes

Liver
Examine for evidence of cirrhosis and any other signs of liver disease

Renal
Check for renal masses

Testes
Examine for testicular masses and groin nodes

AIM: by the end of exam you should have

1. Identified any non-breast pathology which may require investigation/treatment
2. Idea about the grade/extent of gynaecomastia
3. Formulated likely treatment plan

Investigations

- Routine bloods: FBC, U + Es, LFTs, γ-GT
- Special bloods (only if clinical suspicion): TSH, T4, α-fp, testosterone
- Ultrasound (again only if clinical suspicion): thyroid, breast, liver, testes (depending on history/examination)

Treatment

Depends on grade and patient's acceptance of scarring, downtime, etc. with different treatment options (Simon et al. PRS 1973).

Grade	Clinical appearance	Surgical treatment options
Grade 1	Small enlargement (subareolar button) No skin excess	Liposuction alone +/− excision of subareolar excess via periareolar incision
Grade 2a	Moderate enlargement No skin excess	Liposuction alone +/− circumareolar excision of excess tissue (infra-areolar incision = Webster's)
Grade 2b	Moderate enlargement With moderate skin excess	Excision of excess tissue via donut mastopexy technique +/− liposuction to feather edges
Grade 3	Marked enlargement With marked skin excess	Formal breast reduction type technique (type depends on skin excess, i.e., Wise pattern or vertical scar).

Risks/Complications

Early

- Haematoma
- Infection

Late

- Dishing
- Inadequate correction of gland volume or skin excess
- Nipple stuck to chest wall
- Altered nipple sensation
- Obvious scars on male chest wall

Post-operative Management

- Pressure garment (usually cycling vest) for 6 weeks day and night
- Once healed: massage and moisturisation for scars

Further Reading

Fruhstorfer. BJPS 2003. Systematic approach to surgical treatment of gynaecomastia.
Rohrich. PRS 2003. Classification and management of gynaecomastia: defining the role of ulatrsound-assisted liposuction.

Chapter 15
Hand with Nerve Palsy

Shehan Hettiaratchy and Jon Simmons

Focus on addressing specific functional deficits, not trying to recreate all of the nerve's function.

Recognition

Recognise by hand posture:

- Ulnar – hypothenar flat/wasted; little and ring finger claw (MPJ hyperextended +/– flexion of DIPJ/PIPJ depending on high/low lesion) (Fig. 15.1)
- Median – thumb in plane of hand, thenar flat/wasted
- Median and ulnar – both of the above, hand looks flat
- Radial – wrist drop, fingers in flexion

History

General hand
Age, occupation, handedness, hobbies, musical instruments and interference with these.

S. Hettiaratchy (✉)
Department of Plastic and Reconstructive Surgery,
Imperial College Healthcare NHS Trust,
London, UK

S. Hettiaratchy et al. (eds.), *Plastic Surgery*,
DOI 10.1007/978-1-84882-116-3_15,
© Springer-Verlag London Limited 2012

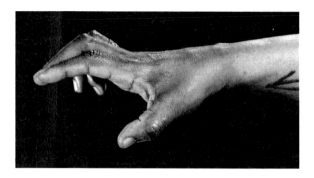

FIGURE 15.1 Hand with nerve palsy

Specific
Cause: trauma or peripheral neuropathy
Time since onset and circumstances
Progression/improvement
Treatment to date both surgical and non-surgical

Current problems:

- Sensory – problems related to loss of sensation; any neuro-pathic pain
- Motor – specific tasks that are difficult

What does the patient hope to gain?

General
Smoking, social setup, support

AIM: by the end of history you should know

1. What the cause was
2. Treatment/progress to date
3. What the patient hopes to achieve
4. Chances of surgery meeting these objectives

Examination

Look
Expose upper limb; scars – supraclavicular/axilla/upper arm/forearm/hand – surgical or traumatic?

Posture
Arm

- Flail: pan-plexus
- Internally rotated: upper root/trunk plexopathy or UMN lesion

Elbow

- Flexed: UMN/central
  - LMN to triceps/plexopathy with radial N
- Flail: C5/6 lesion – upper trunk/root plexopathy/MCN injury

Wrist

- Flexed: Central/UMN
  Radial nerve LMN

Thumb

- Flat median nerve LMN

Fingers

- All flexed: radial nerve
- Ulnar flexed/MCPJ hyperextended (Sign of Benediction) – ulnar nerve palsy
- Little finger abducted – Wartenberg's sign for ulnar nerve

Feel and move
Not a global exam; test specific muscles for specific nerves the confirm with a sensory exam.

Median:
Check sensory (index finger pad) – if PCMN is also involved then lesion is proximal to the wrist.

Anterior Interosseus Nerve:

OK sign – (FPL is anterior interosseous nerve with FDP to index). With an AIN lesion there is no sensory deficit and AbPB is intact. Abductor Pollicis Brevis – test with thumb abduction perpendicular to the palmar plane.

Ulnar:
FCU, FDP to little finger
Interossei (grip paper between fingers without flexing, criss-cross fingers).

Adductor Pollicis (Froment's sign - can they grip paper in 1st web without flexing the thumb IPJ, i.e. using FPL).
Test sensation to little finger. (dorsal branch of ulnar nerve) – if also involved then lesion is proximal to the wrist.

Radial/posterior interosseous nerve (PIN):
Radial nerve – Brachioradialis, Extensor Carpi Radialis Longus/Brevis.
Wrist extensors, finger extensors, Extensor Pollicis Longus. If you find a deficit, try and determine where in the radial nerve/PIN If it is PIN then there is no sensory loss. If there is sensory loss then it is either above the elbow or SBRN. It is – PIN – no sensory loss; – above the elbow. The rest below the elbow therefore after division into PIN. EIP tends to be last branch. Sensory Sensory – first web.

AIM: by the end of exam you should have

1. Identified which nerves are affected
2. Idea about the level of the lesion (high or low)
3. Confirmed what muscles are working for transfer
4. Identified any previous surgery which may impact on your plans

Treatment

The main aim of treatment is to correct deformity and regain specific activities.
These are:

Median: Thumb opposition
    Thumb flexion (if high)
    FDP to index/middle (if high)

Ulnar: Correct claw
    FDP to little/ring (if high lesion)
    Thumb adductor – secondary priority
    Index abductor – secondary priority

Radial: Wrist extension
/PIN Thumb/finger extension

Timing

Non-surgical can be started at any time.

Transfers should only be performed when:
Chance for neurological recovery has passed
Soft tissue is stable and supple
Joints are mobile
Patient is psychologically ready

Options for treatment
Non-surgical

Physiotherapy

• Maintaining passive range of non-motile joints
• Stretching non-innervated muscles
• Softening scars/tissues in preparation for transfer

Splintage

• Helpful for correcting deformity and maintaining joints – preventing capsular/collateral shortening
• Functional splinting (wrist drop) – either static or dynamic

Surgical

Transfers
Remember principles of tendon transfer (APOSLE). May not be able to stick to all of them depending on the clinical situation but more achieved, the better the result.

Median nerve palsy

Opponensplasty: Huber – abductor digiti minimi
                         Bunnell – FDS ring finger
                         Camitz – Palmaris longus
                         Burkhalter – EIP
FPL function: Brachioradialis
FDP to middle/index: Buddy to FDP to ring/little

Ulnar nerve palsy

Claw correction(low):	Need to assess extensor function- if on examination have full extension on correction of the claw then, static procedure may suffice. If extension limited, it will need augmenting with a dynamic transfer
	Static: Zancolli lasso
	Dynamic: ECRL into extensor mechanism using PL as interposition grafts – can use as adductor
Thumb:	Adductor: EIP through palm ?FDS4
FDP to little/ring:	Buddy to FDP index/middle

Radial/PIN

Wrist extensor:	PL to ECRB
Finger extensors:	FCR to EDC
Thumb extensor:	PL to EPL

Risks and Complications

1. Transfer failure
2. Infection
3. Inability to relearn movements

Post-operative Management

1. Immobilise 4-6/52 (protect repairs)
2. Therapy regime (active then passive) to attain transfer function (initiation – get patient to try and reproduce the original function then strengthening/range exercises to increase function)

Outcome

Depends on patient's age and motivation but can get reasonable function. Never as good as the original. Tensioning is extremely important. Some transfers are more forgiving than others.

Chapter 16
Hand with Inflammatory Arthropathy

Shehan Hettiaratchy, Abhilash Jain, and Jon Simmons

Surgery is the last resort once medical treatments have failed but should not be shied away from.

Recognition

Typical arthropathic hand position, splints, walking aids.
Obvious synovitis, previous surgical procedures; scars over MCPJ, CMCJ and dorsal wrist.
Involvement of other joints (neck/shoulders/knees/hips) (Fig. 16.1).

History

General
Age, handedness, occupation, hobbies

Specific
What specific tasks are problematic? 'I can't open jars'

S. Hettiaratchy (✉)
Department of Plastic and Reconstructive Surgery,
Imperial College Healthcare NHS Trust,
London, UK

S. Hettiaratchy et al. (eds.), *Plastic Surgery*,
DOI 10.1007/978-1-84882-116-3_16,
© Springer-Verlag London Limited 2012

117

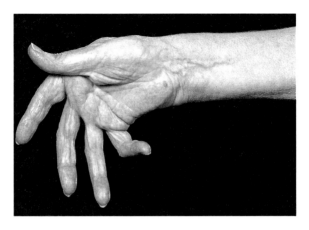

FIGURE 16.1 Hand with arthropathy

What are their specific hand problems? 'I can't straighten my fingers'

What medication are they on, how long have they been on it, who is looking after their arthropathy (GP vs. rheumatologist)

Do they have pain?

Do they have any pins and needles? (occult nerve compressions)

How much of an interference is their hand with normal living? Is it getting worse?

Risk factors

Rheumatoid

Sero-negative arthropathies

Psoriasis

Medication

Current analgesics and anti-inflammatory agents

Current and historic use of: immunosuppressives (e.g., steroids), disease modifying drugs (e.g., methotrexate, gold, sulphasalazine), biological agents (TNF-alpha blockers, e.g., infliximab)

Social

Patients support package and social setup. Will they be able to self-care after an operation.

AIM: by the end of history you should

1. Is there an indication for surgery?
2. What does the patient want to achieve?
3. Are there any other issues that must be addressed first (nerve compression, proximal joint problems, etc)?
4. Have identified any current treatment which would impact on surgical timing, e.g., organising surgery to occur at the midpoint between biological agent doses.

Examination

For efficiency, the examination is broken down into look, feel and move, but combines all three as you work down the upper limb. Before you start remember to ask the patient if any of the joints are painful.

Neck
Bend your neck forwards and back (flexion/extension)
Turn your head to left/right (rotation)

Shoulder
Put your hands behind your head (external rotation and abduction)
Put your hands behind your back and reach up as far as you can on your spine (internal rotation and adduction)

Elbow
Bend your elbows – look/feel for nodules
Straighten your arms
Lock your elbows into your side – turn your palms up and palms down

Wrist
Examine
Dorsal/volar synovitis
Classic wrist deformity – four components

1. Carpal supination (i.e., ulnar side of the wrist has dropped)
2. Volar translocation (carpus has moved volarly)
3. Ulnar translation (carpus has slid down the radius towards the ulna)
4. Radial rotation (compensation for ulnar translation – wrist is radially deviated)

Caput ulnae: prominent ulnar head – compare with other side

Move/feel
Palms together as if you are praying – raise your elbows (extension)
Back of your hands together – push your elbows down (flexion)
Hands out straight, palms down – point them out (ulnar deviation), point them in (radial deviation)
Synovitis
DRUJ piano key-push down on ulna
Check for carpal tunnel syndrome

Thumb and fingers
Look
MPJ–ulnar deviation/volar subluxation/check ulnar intrinsics to see if tight/check EDC to see if subluxed into intermeta-carpal valleys
Fingers – boutonniere or swan neck

Thumb – type of deformity (Nalebuff):

- Type I: Boutonniere, flexed MCPJ
- Type II: Metacarpal adduction with flexed MCPJ
- Type III: Z-shaped thumb/swan neck deformity
- Type IV: CMCJ subluxation due to rupture or attenuation of UCL

Move/feel
Passive joint ranges
Are deformities correctable?
Synovitis
Check extrinsic extensors/flexors (esp. EPL) for ruptures/synovitis

Overview

It may be of benefit to get the patient to demonstrate specific tasks that are difficult as this may make the problem and solution more obvious.

AIM: *by the end of exam you should have*

1. Identified the physical cause of the problem the patient wants addressing
2. Idea of the surgical options and sequence to planned interventions (if any)
3. Idea of the contraindications/prerequisites for surgery
4. Assessed whether the patient is suitable for a surgical inter

Treatment

Operative vs. non-operative

When to treat – Commonly agreed indications for treatment are:

  I. Addressing pain
 II. Improving function
III. Preventative surgery (i.e., synovectomy)
IV. Improving cosmesis

Options for treatment

Non-surgical

Medication

The advent of effective disease modifying medications has had a dramatic effect on our ability to control arthropathies. The monoclonal antibodies have been especially significant. Patients should be managed in a combined fashion with a Rheumatologist.

NO SURGERY SHOULD BE PERFORMED UNTIL MAXIMAL MEDICAL TREATMENT HAS BEEN FOUND TO BE INEFFECTIVE

Splintage

May be helpful for joint flare ups while increased medication is taking time to have an effect.

Hand therapy
Useful to manage symptoms and strengthen the hand within the context of maximising function. Can assess and recommend devices to assist in ADLs.

Surgical
Lots of different options but broadly start with a predictable 'winner'; work proximal to distal and always exclude a nerve compression. Remember that revision procedures are common. Plan incisions accordingly.

1. Synovectomy
2. Joint fusion
3. Joint replacement
4. Tendon transfers
5. Tendon rebalancing

TRIGGER – never release A1 pulley as this will worsen ulnar drift. Triggering in arthropathies is due to synovitis!

Risks and Complications

Tissues very friable
Wound healing worse
Bone healing? worse so need to be meticulous about all bone work
No need to stop steroids and methotrexate
Not clear evidence if anti-TNF must be stopped – arrange surgery mid/late cycle

Post-operative Management

Depends on procedure.
    Ensure adequate support is in place prior to discharge. Plan surgery carefully, staging as necessary to allow patient to continue to cope at home.

Aetiology

Multifactoral, possible environmental factors in susceptible individuals. There is an increased risk in patients with HLA DR1 and HLA DR4. Hormonal influences are also important, during pregnancy disease processes often improve. Flare ups are common in the post-natal period.

Classifications

Several different systems in use for rheumatoid arthritis:

I. By stage
  (a) Stage 1: Proliferative
  (b) Stage 2: Destructive
  (c) Stage 3: Reparative
II. By number of joints affected
  (a) Monoarthropathy
  (b) Pauciarthropathy
  (c) Polyarthropathy
III. By clinical course
  (a) Polycyclic – most common
  (b) Explosive onset
  (c) Progressive
  (d) Monocyclic

Procedures

Arthrodesis
Principles of tendon transfer/reconstruction
Swanson arthroplasty

Controversies

Disease modifying drugs/immunosuppressives/biologics and surgery – should they be stopped?

Chapter 17
Hypospadias

Ivo Gwanmesia and Matthew Griffiths

Hypospadias results from incomplete closure of the urethral folds at 12th week and is characterised by a ventral meatus, hooded foreskin and chordee. It is the most common malformation of the male genitalia with an incidence of 1 in 300 male births.

It can be classified by the meatal position as glanular, coronal, distal, penoscrotal, scrotal or perineal. 70% are distal, 10% mid-penile and 20% the more severe proximal types (Fig. 17.1).

Embryology

3rd week   Primitive streak mesenchymal cells migrate around cloacal membrane to form cloacal folds that fuse cranially to form the genital tubercle

6th week   Cloacal membrane divides into urogenital and anal membranes

Cloacal folds fuse anteriorly – urethral folds

Cloacal folds fuse posteriorly – anal folds

Genital swellings arise lateral to them – labia/scrotal swellings

Pulls urethral folds forwards to form urethral groove

Lining of groove is endodermal (urethral plate)

I. Gwanmesia (✉)
Department of Plastic and Reconstructive Surgery,
Pan-Thames Training Scheme,
London, UK

S. Hettiaratchy et al. (eds.), *Plastic Surgery*,
DOI 10.1007/978-1-84882-116-3_17,
© Springer-Verlag London Limited 2012

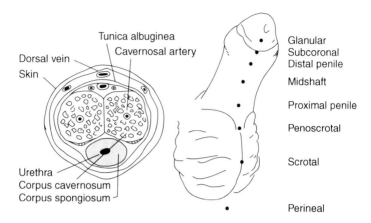

FIGURE 17.1 Classification of hypospadias and penile anatomy

3 months   Urethral folds close over plate to form penile urethra but not into glans
4 months   Distal ectodermal cells migrate into glans as a cord, later to lumenise

Aetiology

Multifactorial

1. Environmental oestrogenic chemicals
2. Androgen hyposensitivity especially with micro penis, undescended testis + inguinal hernia
3. Genetic father–son 8%. Sibs 14%. But not all identical twins, so multifactorial

Recognition

Male child with ventrally placed urethral meatus. Otherwise normal looking child (or adult if delayed presentation).

History

General
Name, age, developmental history, PMH, PSH, DH

Specific

Penis – spraying, stream, witnessed erections
Undescended testes
Groin – inguinal hernia
Renal tract – urinary tract infections and failure to thrive (FTT)
Family history of urogenital problem

AIM: by the end of history you should

1. Have identified the specific issues related to presentation
2. Be aware of family history
3. Have identified any symptoms suggestive of other issues

Examination

General
Normal vs. FTT

Specific

Abdo scars and herniae
Testes
Meatus position
Hooding
Chordee
Depth of urethral groove

AIM: by the end of examination you should

1. Know the position of the meatus
2. Have identified undescended testes and hernia
3. Have identified any previous attempts to correct

Investigations – Not Necessary If Distal

Bedside – Urine dipstick

Bloods – FBC U&Es

Specific – Renal tract USS, urethroscopy, voiding cysto-urethrography

Treatment

Aim to achieve both functional and cosmetic normality

Distal meatal

MAGPI – Duckett (Meatoplasty and glanuloplasty incorporated)

TIP   – Snodgrass (Tubularised incised plate meatoplasty)

Snodgrass (Journal of Urology 1994)

GA + caudal block, anaesthetises mucosa, less bladder spasm, lighter GA, fewer opiates. Gent 7 mg/kg.

Horton erection test – GA, tourniquet, 25 F cannula, 0.9% saline into corpora via glans. Stay suture in glans. Dilate up to 8 F. Remember to follow curve of urethra with dilator. Mark sub-coronal circumferential incision. Leave cuff for circumcision.

Incision carries on below native urethra so it does not retract but rises up with glans once chordee released vertical shaft incision. Chordee lateral to urethra is released and urethra freed up. Lateral skin flaps raised. Check urethra able to reach with urethral plate tubed to end of penis. If more length required will need graft (SnodGraft).

Distal neo-urethra

If ok. Urethral plate incised vertically with bilateral glans incisions to create lateral wall flaps of distal neo-urethra. Dorsal defect re-epithelises with minimal scarring as.

1. Close urethral plate over catheter as first layer – 7/0 polyglactin.
2. Waterproof fascial layer. Inner layer of prepuce can be taken as inner skin and fascia or fascia alone. Based laterally and dissect off prepuce with sharp scissors.

3. Flip over to lateral glans flaps to define terminal meatus. Glans *not* fixated to underlying neourethra. Close with buried 6/0 polyglactin.
4. Close skin with buried 7/0 polyglactin.

Proximal

Bracka – 12 months or at 3 years of age
Bracka does all, does any age, easy to learn, low complication rate.

Bracka – BJU 1995, 76, Suppl. 3, 31–41

For any severity and for any age
Stage 1 – at 3 years of age
GA, tourniquet, 8F catheter, 7 mg/kg dose of gentamicin, Horton erection to test

Sub-coronal incision and dissection to distal corpus cavernous to release chordee. Repeat erection test. Glans split and inner foreskin FTSG or flap to line dorsal aspect of neo-urethra.
Catheter 5 days, EMLA bath or GA change.
Stage 2–6 months after first stage.
NB: Graft mature and soft – needs to be min 15 mm wide with extra 5 mm to be de-epithelised to allow double-breasting.
Prep GA, tourniquet, 8F catheter, dose of gentamicin.
Incision into either side of glans, carried down to form U-shaped incision 15 mm-wide beneath native meatus.
Graft or flap folded over catheter and closed in two layers (Ethilon and PDS).
Third layer derived from foreskin and placed over joint as waterproofing layer.
Circumcision performed as reconstructed foreskin ends up too tight.
Distally, glans flaps closed over catheter.
Lateral skin de-gloved off penis and then closed over as fourth layer.
Post-op – Catheter removed after 1/52.

Complications

Early

Bleeding
Infection
Catheter blockage
Bladder spasm – less with caudal

Intermediate

Fistulae 3%. Early ones due to obstruction, extravasation, haematoma, infection, late due to turbulent flow

Late

Stricture 7%. (2% early. Late mostly due to BXO in FTSG exposed to urine)
Revision 3–5%

Balanitis Xerotica Obliterans – uncommon cause of late strictures – remove all skin graft and replace with buccal mucosa graft – why not do this in the first place? Because it is very difficult to get enough buccal mucosa in the young. Lichen sclerosus (LS) is a chronic, progressive, sclerosing inflammatory dermatosis of unclear etiology. Most reported LS cases (83%) involve the genitalia. In men, this genital involvement has traditionally been known as balanitis xerotica obliterans (BXO). A more accurate term is male genital or penile LS.

Fistulae

Wait for things to settle
Close hole in the urethra
Interpostional fascial flap
Test integrity
NO CATHETER

Follow-Up

Most assessed as normal – 80%
Good urinary function, all forceful stream, 40% spraying
Psyche – 80% confident
83% – straight erections

Chapter 18
Lower Limb Trauma

**Shehan Hettiaratchy, Abhilash Jain,
and Jon Simmons**

Requires joint and simultaneous orthopaedic and plastic surgical management to achieve the best outcome. Amputation can be a good reconstructive option.

Recognition

Treat as a polytrauma using ATLS guidelines. Primary then secondary survey to identify and manage injuries. Initial evaluation and treatment may have to occur simultaneously. External bleeding should be managed with direct pressure.

Beware of high energy injuries (and elderly patients) where zone of injury may not be immediately apparent (Fig. 18.1).

History

In an emergency situation use AMPLE+.
A: Allergies/airway
M: Medications
P : Previous medical/surgical history. PVD, DM, fitness levels

S. Hettiaratchy (✉)
Department of Plastic and Reconstructive Surgery,
Imperial College Healthcare NHS Trust,
London, UK

S. Hettiaratchy et al. (eds.), *Plastic Surgery*,
DOI 10.1007/978-1-84882-116-3_18,
© Springer-Verlag London Limited 2012

131

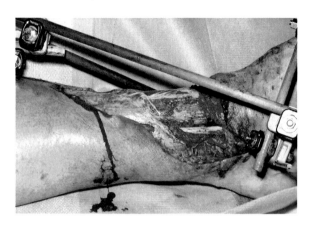

FIGURE 18.1 Lower limb trauma

L: Last meal
E: Event. What are the exact circumstances and nature of the
   trauma. History from first responder gives more detail.
   Consider forces
+: Employment, smoking habits, social circumstances

AIM: by the end of history you should

1. Know the exact mechanism of injury (think compartment
   syndrome)
2. Have an idea of any adverse patient factors (smoking etc.)
3. Have an idea of patient's baseline physical activity/social
   circumstances

Examination

Look
Identify and manage external bleeding. Identify and document all soft tissue, degloving and obvious bony injuries.

*Feel and move. Assess by components and document
findings:*
Skin – Look for degloving; assess by looseness of skin and
viability by blanching/pinprick. Fluorescein is not practical.
Laser doppler can be useful.

Nerves – Test sensation throughout lower limb especially of the sole of the foot – if insensate it may be less urgent to salvage. Outer border of foot (sural n.), dorsum (sup. peroneal n.), 1st web (deep peroneal n.), inner border (saphenous n.), sole (medial and lateral plantar from posterior tibial n.).

Bones/joints – Assess any injured joints for gross instability (within pain limits). XR to assess bony injuries. Views must be complete (joint above and below): AP and Lat.

Exclude an ischaemic limb – surgical emergency. Muscle death begins after 4 h of warm ischaemia. Check pulses by palpation and if not palpable by Doppler compare to an uninjured side. Capillary refill is misleading in the toes. If there is vascular compromise and a non-reduced fracture, reduce the fracture and re-check. If still pulseless proceed to immediate exploration. Do not delay theatre for angiography; level of vascular injury corresponds to fracture site.

Exclude/monitor for a compartment syndrome – surgical emergency. Even in open injuries. Disproportionate pain is the biggest clue, pain on passive movement, tenderness altered sensation. If equivocal, measure all four compartment pressures. Pressure difference between compartment and diastolic of less than 30 mmHg is considered appropriate for decompression.

AIM: by the end of exam you should

1. Have excluded an ischaemic leg and/or compartment syndrome or gross contamination (surgical emergencies)
2. Have an idea about the extent of the soft tissue injury
3. Have an assessment of the bony injury and have adequate imaging of the leg
4. Be ready to photograph, dress and immobilize the limb

Treatment

Immediate treatment
Photograph and then cover the wound with saline soaked gauze and an adhesive film
Immobilize the limb with a splint

IV antibiotics co-amoxiclav 1.2 g or clindamycin if allergic to penicillin

Initial surgical assessment

Done on next trauma list within 24 h of injury unless ischaemic limb or compartment syndrome or gross contamination – immediate. Senior orthopaedic and plastic surgeon. Aims: Sampling of wound for microbiology. Surgical assessment of bone and soft tissue. Aggressive debridement. Perform or plan definitive cover/fixation. It may be possible to achieve definitive fixation and cover in this initial operation (e.g., IM nail/local fasciocutaneous flap).

If more complex reconstruction is required then a temporary external fixator should be put on and the wound(s) dressed with a VAC.

If the limb is non-salvageable it should not be amputated at this sitting unless it poses a risk to the patient. Amputation must be discussed with the patient who should then be given time to consider it, leading to a better psychological outcome.

Intermediate investigations/operations – prepare patient for definitive surgery.

If free flap reconstruction is being planned an angiogram may be required. Consider pre-operative transfusion, filling and warming. CT may be useful for complex or intra-articular fractures.

Further debridements necessary for extensive degloving or contamination. Swabs and samples should be taken each time. Alter antibiotic therapy on the basis of culture results.

Definitive fixation/reconstruction

This is a joint procedure and the end result should be definitive fracture fixation and complete soft-tissue coverage. Numerous options but often involve an Iliziarov/Taylor Spatial Frame with a free flap. Pin site selection is paramount.

Post-operative care

Free flap observations and care. Warming, IVI, FBC, U + E. Close liaison with microbiology for advice about continued antibiotics. DVT prophylaxis is essential. Keep the limb elevated for 5 days and then intermittent lowering to 'stress' the flap and let the venous return improve. Discharge will depend on mobility and weight bearing status.

Follow-up
Required to monitor wound and fracture healing. Frame may be required for 3–4 months, longer for transport procedures.

Outcome

Dependant on injury and treatment
Flap failure 2–4%
Non-union, malunion, delayed union
Osteomyelitis
Amputation
Controversial whether primary amputation or reconstruction gives better long-term results. Should be decided on a case by case basis.

Classifications

Gustillo and Anderson
MESS
AO
Byrd and Spicer
Patterson

Controversies

Amputation vs. reconstruction
Muscle flaps vs. fasciocutaneous flaps
The role of angiography
Timing of reconstruction

Further Reading

Gustillo RB, Anderson, JT. Prevention of infection in the treatment of one thousand and twenty-five open fractures of long bones: retrospective and prospective analyses. J Bone Joint Surg. 1976: 453–458.

Byrd HS: Management of open tibial fractures. Plast Reconstr Surg. 1985;76(5):719–30.

Godina M: Early microsurgical reconstruction of complex trauma of the extremities. Plast Reconstr Surg 1986; 78: 285–92.

Nanchahal J et al: Management of Open Fractures of the Lower Limb. Royal Society of Medicine Press. 2009. Short Guide - http://www.bapras.org.uk/downloaddoc.asp?id=141.

Chapter 19
Lump in the Neck

Farida Ali, Ivo Gwanmesia, and Jon Simmons

A primary tumour can usually be identified in all but 0.5–1%. Patients with positive lymph nodes and an UNKNOWN primary have a better prognosis.

Recognition

Patients often present to the Head and Neck surgeons first, but they always require multidisciplinary input (includes surgeons (ENT/maxillofacial/plastic), pathologist, radiologist, radiotherapist, oncologist, speech therapist, psychologist, clinical nurse specialist and dietician (Fig. 19.1).

History

Age, sex, occupation

General
Cachexia, loss of appetite, weight loss, malaise, pain
Smoker, spices, spirits, poor dentition, drugs (betal nut)

F. Ali (✉)
Department of Plastic and Reconstructive Surgery,
St George's Hospital, London, UK

S. Hettiaratchy et al. (eds.), *Plastic Surgery*,
DOI 10.1007/978-1-84882-116-3_19,
© Springer-Verlag London Limited 2012

137

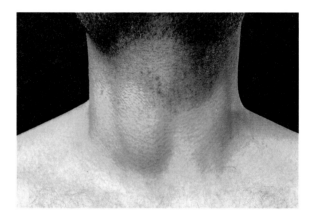

FIGURE 19.1 Patient with lump in the neck

Previous x-ray therapy (e.g., for tinea capitis)
Comorbidities
Social support network

Specific
Intranasal – bleeding, obstruction (usually present late especially post-nasal space)
Intraoral – ulcer, lesion, bleeding, pain, trismus
Pharyngo-oesophageal – dysphagia (solids/liquids)
Laryngeal – dysphonia, hoarseness
Ear – masses, hearing change, discharge, bleeding, pain
Salivary glands – swelling, pain
Neck – thyroid, parathyroid mass
Respiratory – cough, haemoptysis, SOB
Upper GIT – dyspepsia, dysphagia, pain
Other, e.g., lymphoma – Other masses elsewhere?
Skin, pigmented/non-pigmented lesions, sun exposure etc. as for skin cancer, e.g., scalp

Examination

Be systematic
Use a pen torch and tongue depressor for the intraoral examination (if you do not have one, ASK)

General

General status of patient (note presence of signs of advanced CA? – cachexia, anaemia etc.)

Other lymph node basins (lymphoma)

Other systems (respiratory, GI)

Specific

Look

Is there an obvious mass? Single or multiple, midline or lateral?

Extraoral – lip, external nose, ear, skin, scalp. Look for any obvious lesions.

Intraoral – mucosa, alveolar ridges, tongue, palate, floor of mouth, pharyngeal, tonsils – Looking for masses, ulceration, leukoplakia, blood from Stenson's duct (opposite upper second molar).

Intranasal – using a nasal speculum look for any masses on both sides.

Salivary gland masses, blood at Stenson's duct orifice.

Palpation

Neck – clearly demonstrate each level to the examiner. Involved level can give an indication to potential primary sites. Identify whether single node or multiple and matted nodes. With midline masses, identify presence of movement with swallowing or tongue protrusion.

If there are any suspicious lesions from your inspection, then examine them.

Intraoral – use gloves and digitally palpate the mucosa, alveolar ridges, floor of mouth and tongue. Look for blood at the opening of Stenson's duct on palpation of the parotid gland(s).

Aim: By the end of the history and examination, you should have

1. Narrowed down your likely primary sites (although investigations are required to rule out synchronous/multiple system tumours)

2. Identified the level and laterality of involved lymph node(s)
3. Made an assessment of the general status of the patient including fitness for surgery

Investigations

1. CXR and OPG
2. Further imaging. This should be done BEFORE biopsy for two reasons. First, it guides biopsy of identified suspicious areas and secondly, interpretation will not be compromised by postoperative oedema.
   - *MRI scan* (Head and Neck)
     Primary lesion peri tumour oedema on T2 weighted images. Estimate size, extent, invasion of neighbouring structures (all required to stage the disease)
   - *CT Head and Neck*
     Good for bony lesions/ bony invasion
   - *PET Scan/PET-CT*
     More sensitive than CT or MRI
     Can be superimposed onto CT to identify whether a mass on CT and enhancing area on PET scan correspond
3. FNAC: If non-specific, repeat once more. If still inconclusive, then open biopsy (scar placement should allow incorporation into neck dissection access incisions).
4. Panendoscopy: Any abnormal site (clinical or radiographic) should be biopsied. IN ADDITION, always biopsy nasophayrnx, tonsils, piriform fossa, base of tongue and floor of mouth.

Suspicious Lymph nodes on MRI/CT
>0.5 cm
Central necrosis
Loss of architecture
Extracapsular spread
Multiple or matted nodes

Treatment

Known primary
Treatment dictated by histopathological diagnosis and a multidisciplinary discussion of each case. May be non-surgical, surgical or combined.

Unknown primary
Nodal cytology/histology may guide you somewhat.
Squamous cell carcinoma – more likely head and neck/skin origin
Adenocarcinoma – more likely lung, breast, GI malignancy

Treatment of Likely Primary Sites
Unilateral/ bilateral tonsillectomy – Controversial. Occult tonsillar carcinoma seen in up to 40% cases (McQuone et al. 1998).

Radiotherapy to potential sites – Controversial. Likewise, unilateral or bilateral treatment is also debatable. Suggestion that bilateral radiotherapy to potential primary sites shows better disease control, particularly with bilateral lymphadenopathy; however, some studies show increase in local control but no change in overall survival (Mahoney Otolaryngologic Clinics 2005).

TNM definitions for oral cavity and oropharynx
TX: cannot assess primary tumour
T0:   no evidence of primary tumour
Tis: carcinoma in situ
T1:   tumour <2 cm
T2:   tumour 2–4 cm
T3:   tumour >4 cm
T4:   tumour invades adjacent structures

N1:   single, ipsilateral /unilateral, <3 cm
N2a: single, ipsilateral/unilateral, 3–6 cm
N2b: multiple ipsilateral/unilateral, <6 cm
N2c: contralateral/bilateral, <6 cm
N3:   any lymph node, >6 cm

MX: distant metastases cannot be assessed
M0: no distant metastases
M1: distant metastases

Treatment of the Neck

This depends on the stage of the disease

N0 neck

Neck dissection not performed for T1 tumours. Neck dissection is performed for T2, T3 and T4 tumours

N positive neck – Neck dissection is performed for N positive necks

N1/N2a

Single Modality Treatment

Neck dissection alone or radiotherapy alone (after excision of node). However, if extracapsular spread or multiple nodes are confirmed on histology, postoperative radiotherapy is usually recommended.

N2b/2c/3

Combined Treatment

A combination of neck dissection and radiotherapy is generally accepted. However, still controversial whether radiotherapy should be neo-adjuvant or adjuvant.

Chemotherapy. Mixed results reported with chemotherapy, but usually recommended for inoperable disease or in the presence of distant metastases.

Surgical Management of the Neck

Known primary – dictates whether selective or modified radical ND is indicated

Unknown primary – usually indicates modified radical ND

Chapter 20
Complex Wounds: Pressure Sore

Jon Simmons and Matthew Griffiths

The last thing to consider in pressure sore management is the wound. Need to optimise all other factors first. Surgery rarely indicated.

Recognition

Consider pressure areas relative to the individual patient. Elderly bed-bound patient vs. young patient in a wheelchair. Approximately 3% of hospitalised patients have a pressure sore (Fig. 20.1).

Pathophysiology

Capillary arterial circulation will cease with pressures greater than 32 mmHg, 8–10 mmHg for venous capillary network. Constant pressure for >2 h produces irreversible changes. Muscle is more susceptible than skin. Ischial tuberosities are exposed to 100 mmHg when seated, when supine, occiput, heel and sacrum are exposed to 50 mmHg. Bacterial growth

J. Simmons (✉)
Department of Plastic and Reconstructive Surgery,
Imperial College Healthcare NHS Trust,
London, UK

S. Hettiaratchy et al. (eds.), *Plastic Surgery*,
DOI 10.1007/978-1-84882-116-3_20,
© Springer-Verlag London Limited 2012

143

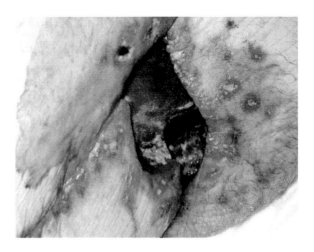

FIGURE 20.1 Wound breakdown in a pressure area

also increased in pressure areas due to ischaemia, impaired lymphatics and impaired immune function. Neurological injury further decreases local tissue perfusion due to local tissue oedema. Dilution of sebum concentrations reduces its anti-staph and anti-strep activity. Shear forces.

History

When and where, how long, getting better/worse, problems, current dressing management, devices, previous surgery, changes in circumstances (for instance a patient who has spent a long time in bed on ITU who has recovered and is now mobile) and prognosis.

General health

CNS/PNS	Level of injury, CVA, MS
CVS	Arteriopath, anaemia, BP, cholesterol,
RS	COPD, asthmatic (suitability for general anaesthesia)
GIT	Nutrition, stoma, incontinence
GUS	Renal function, incontinence
Endo	DM, thyroid
MS	Skin quality, joint problems, mobility

Surgical/medical/medicines history – Previous surgery for pressure sores, medication, immunosuppression with medicines or illness, smoking.

Social history – Occupation, partner, care package, home modifications, pressure relieving devices.

AIM: by the end of history you should have

1. Understood the ulcer's aetiology and history along with the patient's likely prognosis
2. Any adverse patient factors (BMI, immobility, immuno-compromise, infection, smoking)
3. Understood whether any causative or adverse patient factors can be reversed

Examination

Consider Waterlow Score for ulcer prevention

General – Age, sex, mobility, nutrition, position and posture, pressure relief (cushions etc.) General health of the patient, anaemia, cachexia.

Wound and surrounding skin quality – size, edges, base, surface. Areas affected in decreasing frequency; ischium (30%), sacrum (20%), trochanter (15%) and the heel (10%). Remember the extent of underlying muscle damage is greater than that of the overlying skin.

Only now consider staging!

Staging: NPUAP – National Pressure Ulcer Advisory Panel

  I: Non-blanchable intact skin
 II: Superficial partial skin loss, blistering
III: Full-thickness skin loss and subcutaneous destruction into muscle
IV: Involvement of bone/joint

AIM: by the end of examination you should

1. Understand the site involved and the aetiology in this particular individual

2. Understand the extent of the soft tissue/bony defect and be ready to describe the stage of the ulcer
3. Made an assessment of the general health of the patient and any reversible factors
4. Have understood any previous surgical interventions (with respect to donor sites already used – some flaps may be readvanced)

Management: Prevention Is the Key

Patient: Nutrition
Involve dietician – Build up drinks, adequate intake, enteral or parenteral feeding may be appropriate. Robson et al. demonstrated normal healing if albumin above 20. Consider vitamin and mineral supplements in the form of Vitamin A and C (required for normal wound healing), Zinc (epithelialisation and fibroblast proliferation) and calcium (co-factor for many enzymes).

Patient/Nursing – Pressure
Dinsdale (Arch Phys Med Rehab 1974) demonstrated the ability to negate pressure by relieving for 5 min every 2 h. Pressure when seated is higher than supine and so relief should be more frequent.

Patient – Continence
Catheterise and consider stoma if large perianal wound.

Patient – Spasticity
Diazepam 10 mg every 8 h
Baclofen 10 mg every 6 h
Dantrolene 25 mg every 12 h

Nursing – different mattresses for increasing risk (based on Waterlow score)
Foam
Static flotation
Alternating air
Low air loss
Air fluidised, e.g., clinitron

Surgery: General Principles

1. Patient selection is of paramount importance – most sores can be managed non-operatively with pressure relief, patient optimisation, manual sharp debridement and careful wound care
2. Excisional debridement of ulcer, bursa and heterotopic calcification
3. Partial/complete osteotomy/osteoectomy reduce bony prominence
4. Closure with healthy padded tissue

Debridement
Limited debridement can be performed on the ward to deroof the necrotic tissue.

Theatre
Place in position so wound given maximal exposure and therefore flaps positioned at minimal tension post-op. This should reduce wound dehiscence post-op. Aggressive excision of wound – tumour type.

Osteoectomy
Removal of bony prominences required.

Radical excision of bone redistributes pressure to other areas, causes excessive bleeding and skeletal instability.

Ischial ulcers. Total ischectomies reduce recurrence rate from 38% to 3% but contralateral ulcers formed in one-third of patients.

Bilateral ischectomies move pressure to perineum which can complicate to the formation of urethral fistulas.

Primary closure
Always leaves a subcutaneous space.

SSG
30% success is associated with this technique.

Musculocutaneous flaps
Mathes demonstrated theoretical advantage of muscle flaps. Excellent blood supply, bulky padding and can be re-advanced or re-rotated. However muscle is the most sensitive to ischaemic injury, may be atrophic in the elderly and spinal patients or lead to functional disability in ambulatory patients.

Fasciocutaneous flaps
Offer adequate blood supply, durable coverage with minimal potential for a functional deformity and more closely reconstruct the normal anatomic arrangement over bony prominences. Limited tissue available for the treatment of large ulcers.

Outcome

Dependant on many factors
Recurrence rates are high
Complications include: haematoma, seroma, infection and wound dehiscence

Classifications

National Pressure Ulcer Advisory Panel staging system
Waterlow Scoring System

Procedures

Sacral sores – buttock rotation flaps (musculocutaneous or fasciocutaneous)
Trochanteric sores – TFL, Vastus lateralis, ALT
Ischial sores – hamstrings muscle flap, posterior thigh flap

Controversies

Operative vs. non-operative management
Musculocutaneous vs. fasciocutaneous flaps. Which is better?

Chapter 21
Abnormal Ear

**Ivo Gwanmesia, Matthew Griffiths,
and Jon Simmons**

Abnormal ears are either congenital or acquired. Congenital types may either be prominent ears suitable for correction or may be more severe and be part of a syndrome and require reconstruction. Acquired ear deformities are usually secondary to trauma.

Recognition

Young patient presenting with parents or adult usually male following trauma. Young adults may present with prominent ears where parents have resisted/deferred seeking treatment for their child (Fig. 21.1).

Embryology

Ear forms between weeks 4 and 8
6 auricular hillocks form around the 1st branchial groove
1–3 form from the 1st arch and form tragus, root and superior helix
4–6 posteriorly from 2nd arch and form rest of helix, anti-helix, scapha, antitragus and lobule and triangular fossa

I. Gwanmesia (✉)
Department of Plastic and Reconstructive Surgery,
Pan-Thames Training Scheme,
London, UK

S. Hettiaratchy et al. (eds.), *Plastic Surgery*,
DOI 10.1007/978-1-84882-116-3_21,
© Springer-Verlag London Limited 2012

FIGURE 21.1 Abnormal ear

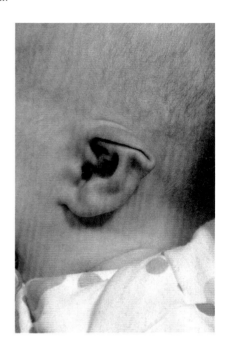

FIGURE 21.1 Abnormal ear

History

Prominent ears

Was deformity present at birth?
Are there any hearing problems?
Is the child being teased at school?
Does the child feel that his/her ear is a problem?
Are there any other abnormalities?

Congenital
History similar as above.

More emphasis on hearing status and the presence of other anomalies if suspicion of congenital cause.

If more severe then relevant paediatric history. Family history.

Traumatic ears
Previous debridements, replantation or attempts at reconstruction

AIM: by the end of history you should have

1. Identified any other conditions which may influence surgical management
2. Understood the reasons that treatment are sought at this point in the child's life – who is driving the process
3. Traumatic – Identified any previous attempts to resolve the problem

Examination

Prominent ears

Assess upper third	– Defined by presence of anti-helical fold
Assess middle third	– Defined by depth of conchal bowl
Assess lower third	– Size of lobule
Comment on symmetry	– Which side is more projected

Lateral protrusion of helix from head ranges from 17 to 21 mm (normal)

Congenital/traumatic

- Any other congenital anomalies, facial asymmetry
- Quality of surrounding skin
- Previous incisions and skin grafts
- Type of microtia – conchal or lobular
- Size of costal margin (for rib grafting 58–60 cm circumference required as a minimum)
- Hairline in relation to projected position (important not to have hair on the helical rim)
- Extent of defect – what will be required for reconstruction in terms of partial or complete framework
- Ear problems common in Treacher–Collins (mandibulofacial dysostosis), Goldenhar and hemifacial microsomia, but often sporadic

AIM: by the end of examination you should have

1. Assessed the suitability of the patient for surgery
2. Identified other congenital anomalies that might influence surgery or timing of surgery

3. Formulated a surgical plan and timeline
4. Identified any factors which might require treatment prior to definitive surgery, e.g., laser to raise a hairline

Management

Neonates (Ear buddies)

More pliable cartilage, do not sweat, cannot reach ear, splint for 2/52.
If more than 1/12 splint for 3/52.
Matsuo managed the correction of congenital auricular deformities in 150 patients using various moulds and tapes to achieve correction.
Cartilage is uniquely mouldable in the first 6 weeks of life due to maternal hormones.

Congenital – Microtia

About 90 cases per year/UK sub-specialised field, few surgeons doing large numbers.
85% of ear growth done by 3 years of age, but insufficient costal cartilage until at least 6 years of age.
Ear height continues into the adulthood.

Options

1. *Prosthetic reconstruction*
   (a) Adhesive
   (b) Branemark
2. *Autologous/alloplastic reconstruction*
   Medpore implant with local temporoparietal fascial flap (TPF) and SSG
3. *Autologous reconstruction*
   Costal cartilage with local temporoparietal fascial flap and SSG

Tanzer 1959 Six stage technique
Brent 1974 Four stage technique – pocket, lobe transposition, lift ear, tragus
Nagata 1985 Two stage technique – most practiced in the UK

- *Framework constructed using rib held and positioned with steel sutures and shaped. Depending on the defect a floating rib is used for the helix and a rib block formed from the syndesmosis is used to form the remaining structure. Pocket dissected and framework inserted with tragus premade using the pedicled transposed lobe. A left over block is banked in a subcutaneous pocket usually on the abdomen, to be used in the second stage.*
- *After a minimum of 6/12. Elevate framework with costal cartilage in the sulcus. TPF or fascial flap and SSG from occipital scalp to resurface the sulcus.*

Hearing

Inner ear develops from different arches so tends to be present. Bone anchored hearing aids (BAHA) work but need to be positioned sensitively so that local reconstructive options are not affected.

Traumatic ears

Options

1. Nothing
2. Prosthesis as above
3. Autologous/alloplastic reconstruction as above
4. Replantation. Rarely successful. Small artery, unlikely to find a suitable vein and may suffer catastrophic fall in Hb due to leeching

Prominent ears

If very early then may be able to avoid surgery with 'ear buddies' when cartilage is mouldable.

The current trend is more for suture based techniques rather than full degloving of ear, scoring or cartilage excision, accepting a slightly higher revision rate but much less severe complications.

1. If less severe prominent ear in younger child then consider degloving of posterior pinna, with or without fascial flap and then around three *scapho-conchal* horizontal mattress of PDS or Ethibond on a round bodied needle to recreate more normal, rounded anti-helical fold. Then dissect small

pocket in retroauricular area and use similar *concho-mastoid* sutures to set and posteriorly rotate the whole pinna.
2. If more severe then may need to consider posterior scoring or classic Chongchet 1963 BJPS cartilage excision and anterior scoring – rarely necessary.

Miscellaneous

Normal ear characteristics

1. Ear position usually one ear length from lateral orbital rim
2. 6.5–7.5 cm length
3. Width = 55% of length
4. Conchal bowl 1.5 cm deep
5. Top of ear in line with brow
6. Bottom of ear in line with base of columella

Ear anatomy

Need to be able to define all the parts.
Helical rim, scapha, anti-helical fold, concha, superior and inferior crura, triangular fossa, cymbum concha, cavum concha, tragus, antitragus, lobule, helical root (Fig. 21.2).

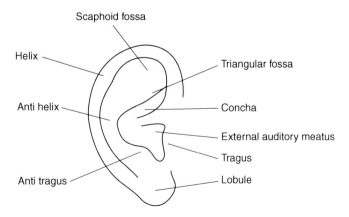

FIGURE 21.2 Normal ear anatomy

Tanzer classification of auricular defects

1. Anotia
2. Microtia
    (a) Atresia of EAM
    (b) Without atresia of the EAM
3. Hypoplasia of the middle third of the auricle
4. Hypoplasia of the superior third of the auricle
    (a) Constricted (cup or lop) ear
    (b) Cryptotia
    (c) Hypoplasia of the entire superior third

McDowell outlined the basic goals – prominent ears

1. Correct all protrusion of the upper third of the ear
2. From the front, helix of both ears should be beyond anti-helix
3. Smooth helix
4. Post-auricular sulcus should not be decreased or distorted
5. Outer helix to mastoid
    (a) Top 10–12 mm
    (b) Middle 16–18 mm
    (c) Lower 20–22 mm
6. Position of the ear should be within 3 mm of each other

Chapter 22
Management of the Pigmented Lesion

Fiona Harper

Melanoma: Tumour of epidermal melanocytes. Should be managed in multi-disciplinary team setting: dermatologist, surgeon, pathologist, oncologist, clinical nurse specialist. Increasing prevalence in UK. Managed initially by local skin cancer MDTs (LSMDTs) core services and referred to specialist skin cancer MDTs (SSMDTs).

Recognition

Elderly patient with Fitzpatrick 1 or 2 presenting with obvious sun damaged skin. Younger patient with fair skin with history of excessive sun exposure. Patient with Fitzpatrick 4, 5 or 6 with a lesion on the sole of the foot or subungally (Fig. 22.1).

History

General introduction
2 week rule

F. Harper
Specialist Registrar in Plastic and Reconstructive Surgery,
Pan-Thames Training Scheme,
London, UK

S. Hettiaratchy et al. (eds.), *Plastic Surgery*,
DOI 10.1007/978-1-84882-116-3_22,
© Springer-Verlag London Limited 2012

157

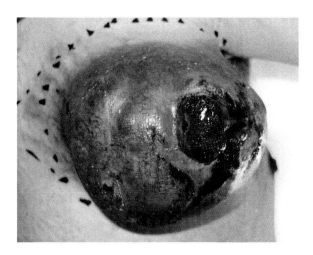

FIGURE 22.1 Lymph node melanoma metastasis with unknown primary

Urgent referral to LSMDT if:

- New mole appearing after onset of puberty with change in shape/colour/size
- Longstanding mole with change in shape/colour/size
- Any mole with more than three colours, loss of symmetry
- Itching/bleeding
- Persistent skin lesion growing/pigmented/vascular appearance

General
Age, occupation, hobbies, previous and current sun exposure
Full medical and drug history

Specific
Duration of lesion
Change in

- Size
- Shape
- Colour
- Itching/bleeding

Risk factors (melanoma)

Moderately increased risk (8–10×)	Atypical mole phenotype Previous melanoma Organ transplant
Greatly increased risk (>10×)	Giant congenital pigmented hairy naevus FH x 3 or more cases of melanoma Pancreatic carcinoma

AIM: by the end of the history you should know

1. Duration and characteristics of lesion
2. Risk factors for melanoma
3. General medical factors that may influence management

Examination

Look/feel

- Site
- Size
- Elevation
- Description
- Other pigmented lesions
- Regional lymph nodes
- Hepatomegaly

Plus: Complete skin examination including Fitzpatrick skin type
+/− dermatoscopy
Photography

AIM: by the end of the examination you should know

1. Macroscopic features of the lesion and other lesions
2. Clinical evaluation of the presence of secondary disease
3. General skin quality/evidence of sun exposure

Biopsy of Suspected Melanoma

Photograph first
Full thickness, including the whole tumour, 2 mm lateral margin plus cuff of fat
Incisional biopsy occasionally acceptable (e.g. lentigo maligna)

Subungal melanoma:

Biopsy by surgeons regularly doing so. Important to biopsy germinal matrix.
Removal of sufficient nail plate + any clinically obvious tumour.

Investigations

Stage l and ll
Routine investigation not required

NICE guidelines
Patients should be offered sentinel lymph node biopsy (SLNB) if their tumour is: Stage lB and upwards (<1 mm, with ulceration or mitoses or >1 mm

Stage lll (Lymph node involvement)
CT head/chest/abdomen/pelvis

Stage lV (Metastic disease)
CT head + consider whole body
Serum LDH

Treatment/Surgical Technique

Of primary tumour
Wide local excision (WLE)

Breslow thickness in situ/lentigo maligna	5 mm
<1 mm	1 cm
1.01–2 mm	1–2 cm

| 2.01–4 mm | 2–3 cm |
| >4 mm | 3 cm |

Of lymph node basins

Clinically node –ve	SNLB
	Performed at same time as WLE
Clinically or radiologically suspicious nodes	FNAC repeat if –ve or US-guided core biopsy
	Open biopsy
Confirmed + ve lymph node metastases	Axillary LND Levels l–lll
	Superficial Inguinal LND
	Pelvic LND
	Cervical LND – comprehensive

LND should only be performed by SSMDT members who do AT LEAST 15 LNDs for skin cancer/year

Options for treatment of locoregional recurrence

Single local or regional metastasis	Surgery	
Multiple local metastases	CO_2 laser ablation	
Regional chemotherapy	Isolated limb infusion	3 UK centres
	Isolated limb perfusion	2 UK centres
Electrochemotherapy	Novel treatment. Relies on electroporation using an intralesional electrode to damage melanoma cells and make them more susceptible to intralesional or systemic bleomycin	
Adjuvant therapy	No evidence of a survival benefit	

Occult primary melanoma:

May present with solitary metastasis/lymph node/systemic disease

Prompt referral to SSMDT – thorough examination: skin/uveal tract/genital/urinary tracts/anorectum

All patients should be staged with CT head/chest/abdo/pelvis

Treatment should be appropriate to the tumour regardless of the inability to detect the primary

Risks/Complications

General
Risks of LA
GA: DVT/PE/Chest infection

Specific
Following LND: Damage to nerves/vessels, infection, poor wound healing wound dehiscence, exposure of vital structures, seroma, lymhoedema

Post-operative Management

Follow-up rationale	Detect recurrence
	Detect further primaries
	Support/information/education
In situ	No follow up
Stage 1A	2–4 visits for 1 year
Stage IB–IIIA	5 years
Stage (IIIB–IIIC+	10 years
Resected stage IV)	
Unresectable stage IV	Seen according to need

Prevention

Avoid sunburn
Avoid sunbed usage

Papers to Know

Revised UK guidelines for the management of cutaneous melanoma 2010. British Association of Dermatology.

2009 AJCC Melanoma Staging and Classification
Charles M. Balch, Jeffrey E. Gershenwald, Seng-jaw Soong, John F. Thompson, Michael B. Atkins, David R. Byrd, Antonio C. Buzaid, Alistair J. Cochran, Daniel G. Coit, Shouluan Ding, Alexander M. Eggermont, Keith T. Flaherty, Phyllis A. Gimotty, John M. Kirkwood, Kelly M. McMasters, Martin C. Mihm Jr, Donald L. Morton, Merrick I. Ross, Arthur J. Sober and Vernon K. Sondak Journal of Clinical Oncology.

Veronesi New England Journal of Medicine 1988

- No difference between 1 and 3 cm margins for MM < 2 mm deep

Balch Annals of Surgery 1995

- 2 cm excision adequate for MM 1–4 mm deep

WHO Lancet 1998

- No benefit from ELND

Morton   NEJM   2006   (Multicenter   Selective Lymphadenectomy Trial data)

- For MM 1–4 mm SLNB useful for staging and prolongs disease free interval
- Improved survival for patients undergoing CLND for micromets
- No increase in local or intransit mets after SLNB
- Support for micromets becoming macro or distant disease

Chapter 23
Aged Face: Facelifting

Shehan Hettiaratchy

The key to success of facial rejuvenation is to refresh the patient while maintaining facial harmony, i.e., they should STILL look normal and not Picasso-esque.

Recognition

Middle aged women and less commonly men but increasingly older and younger patients are presenting (Fig. 23.1).

History

General introduction – Age, occupation, hobbies, smoking, sun exposure

Specific

- Start with an open question 'How can I help?' and let the patient voice their areas of concern
- How long have they been considering facial rejuvenative surgery?
- Which areas particularly bother them?

S. Hettiaratchy
Department of Plastic and Reconstructive Surgery,
Imperial College Healthcare NHS Trust,
London, UK

S. Hettiaratchy et al. (eds.), *Plastic Surgery*,
DOI 10.1007/978-1-84882-116-3_23,
© Springer-Verlag London Limited 2012

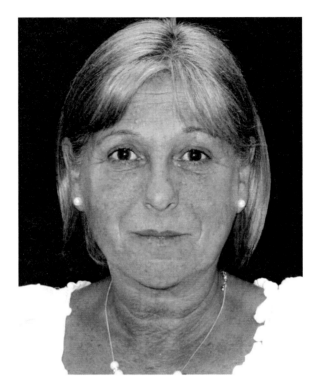

FIGURE 23.1 Patient presenting for facial rejuvenation

- What kind of appearance do they want? Do they want to look refreshed or significantly younger?
- Have they had any rejuvenative procedures in the past?
- Do they know anyone who has had this type of surgery?
- How much time off do they envisage having, i.e., how much 'downtime' will they accept?
- Who is at home? Where will they convalesce?
- Do they have any specific deadlines/events at which they must be presentable?

Risk factors

- Smoking
- Medications (aspirin, NSAIDs, herbal medications, anticoagulants – all increase the risk of bleeding)

- Bleeding tendencies
- Hypertension
- Previous facial surgery

General

- Full health questionnaire including cardiac/respiratory history
- Medications and allergies
- Previous surgery and general anaesthesia
- Suggest an anaesthetic assessment if required

AIM: by the end of history you should

1. Have an idea of the problem areas the patient wishes to address and their expectations
2. Have an idea of how much downtime they are willing to accept
3. Have assessed their medical fitness for a procedure
4. Have identified any with unrealistic aims – red flags

Examination

Look

This is the part where people get stumped. The typical changes with aging are brow ptosis, eye changes, midface ptosis (with uncovering of the bony skeleton, deepening of the NLF and jowling with skin bunching up and hanging down lateral and below the NLF), and neck laxity. Jowling leads to the face changing from a youthful oval to a more squared appearance. This can be attractive in a man but makes women look sad and sour. People talk about the 'ogee' which is the shape the full cheek makes when seen in half profile. This is lost in aging. The chin can also ptose, adding to the older face appearing longer and the neck will have developed folds of loose skin (turkey gobbler neck). In addition there is loss of cervico-mental angle when seen in profile.

The best way is to make a quick overall assessment of their skin, hair and general appearance. Make specific note of any asymmetries and point these out to the patient.

Next work through the face in areas thinking in terms of the procedures that can be performed and if the patient needs them. This should lead to a surgical menu for the patient that can be used depending on how extensive the surgery they want is and how rich they are feeling.

General assessment

Assess the skin – is there sun damage, lots of wrinkles (rhytids) and are they fine or coarse, i.e., does the patient need some form of resurfacing/fillers/botox?

Look at the hair – is it thin, thick, receding, i.e., can you hide scars easily in there? Can you move the hairline?

Is their face thin – will they need volume added with fat transfers? Look particularly at lips, NLF, malars, chin as these areas can all look good with some gentle augmentation.

Specific

It is somewhat artificial to think of the face in strict thirds. Think of it as areas to be addressed.

Upper – brow

Midface – eyes, nose, midface comprising cheek, naso-labial fold and jowl (these will be addressed by midface lifting)

Central/lower – mouth/perioral, chin, neck.

Upper

- Do they have lateral brow ptosis with hooding and heaviness? They may need a browlift (usually endobrow but this tends to work best in females). Brow position.
- Have they got marked glabellar lines? This would benefit from botox.

Midface

- Do they need something to be done to their eyes? Do they need upper blephs? Do they need lower blephs? (See chapter on blepharoplasties)

- How much midface ptosis is there? See how much skeletal show there is (especially along the infraorbital margin), how deepened the NLF are due to cheek overhang, and how much jowling they have; all of these can be improved by midface lifting.
- Nose – should you mention it? Do they need a rhinoplasty? (see chapter on rhinoplasty) This will not contribute to making them look younger but may improve the overall aesthetics of their face. You may not wish to raise it unless they comment on it.

Central/Lower

- Are their lips thin? Do they need augmentation with fillers/fat transfer/dermal fat graft?
- Do they have perioral rhytids (called bleed lines as lipstick 'bleeds' into them)? Do they have marionette lines (vertical lines either side of the mouth)? Would these benefit from resurfacing or fillers?
- Do they have chin ptosis or a weak chin? Would it benefit from augmentation/advancing?
- Do they have neck laxity with excess skin? Do they have platysmal bands (midline divarification of the anterior edges of the platsyma – can be addressed by lateral platysmaplasty but may need direct division of the bands to soften)? Is there loss of the cervico-mental angle? This can be addressed with submental liposuction and lateral platysmaplasty which should tighten the neck, give a clean jawline and redefine the cervio-mental angle.

Finally, make an assessment as to whether they would benefit from volume addition (e.g., fat transfers). Look particularly at lips, NLF, malars, chin.

Make sure you check in front and behind the ears for scars from previous procedures; patients often 'forget' that they have had work before!

B) Feel/move
This is time to employ the 'magic' finger to move the soft tissues to get an idea of what surgery can achieve. Try and use

the same vectors as would occur with the surgical gestures but explain to the patient that surgery will not do exactly the same as the finger manipulation. Reproduce the endobrow, midface lift and neck lift. As well as demonstrating to the patient what may be achieved, you can assess whether they will need volume added as well as the lifting procedures.

Finally, check the function of cranial nerves V and VII.

AIM: by the end of exam you should

1. Have an idea of what the patient wants
2. Have an idea of if and how you can deliver it

Investigations

FBC, U&Es, clotting
Photographs

Treatment

Facelift surgery is complicated by lots of different terminology so it is important to get back to the basics. The aim of face lift surgery is to reposition any ptosed soft tissues (e.g., fat pockets) and tighten skin that has lost elastic recoil.

It is not possible to tighten fat, so facelifts work by tightening fascia that contains the fat and moves it back to its original place.

There are three layers that can be moved to reposition the soft tissues of the face:

1. Skin
2. SMAS (superficial musculo-aponeurotic system)
3. Periosteum

All facelifts use one, two or all of these layers. The most common one used is the SMAS that can be tightened in various ways.

Skin only
Rarely performed but was the mainstay until 1980s. Possible indication would be a skin only problem, but most facelifts now involve some form of SMAS manipulation.

SMAS procedures
SMAS is the modern workhorse of facelifting. Pulling on the SMAS repositions the malar fat pad, decreases the overhang on the NLF, corrects jowling and also addresses the neck. SMAS can either be:

• Left in situ and tightened with sutures (plication)
• Part of the mobile SMAS is excised along an oblique line and sutured onto the immobile SMAS (SMASectomy)
• SMAS is elevated as a flap and any excess trimmed off (SMAS flaps)

Periosteal procedures

• These can be very powerful ways of moving the soft tissues on the bony skeleton. This may be indicated in a redo face-lift (advantage of a fresh plane) or when trying to correct lower lid/lateral canthal malposition.
• Various different access options including bicoronal, lower lid and buccal sulcal.
• Mask lift is a pure periosteal procedure done via a bicoronal approach.
• The downside is the invasiveness of the surgery and the time to recover.

Composite Rhytidectomy

• Skin and SMAS are dissected as a composite
• Flap is less likely to slough
• Extensive procedure

Neck procedures

Corset platysmaplasty
Submental dissection and platysmaplasty
Plastysma flaps
Liposuction

Adjuncts to face lifting
Brow-lifting

This is often performed in female patients and addresses not just the brow but also the forehead and temple. Usually done endoscopically, but the patient must have a short forehead (7 cm) and it must not be overly curved.

3 or 5 port techniques are described and there are various means of fixation.

Advantage of the browlift is that it opens up the eyes especially laterally.

Fat transfers

Adds volume to the face to regain youthful contours and fullness.

Fillers

Fill out fine rhytids around the mouth and redefine the vermillion border.

Resurfacing

Addresses fine rhytids and also causes some tightening. The available methods are chemical peeling, laser resurfacing and dermabrasion. Each surgeon will have a preference for a method and no one method has been shown to be better than another.

Botulinum toxin type-A

Can be used to deal with glabellar lines, crows' feet.

Can also be used for contralateral symmetrization for a unilateral marginal mandibular branch palsy.

Post-operative Management

- Sit up post-op for 24 h; sleep at 45°
- Drains (either Penrose or small lantern) reduce bruising and swelling but not haematomas
- Firm dressing of jelonet/gauze/wool/crepe for 24 h, then no dressings

- Remove dressings and wash hair before discharge
- Gentle mobilization but no straining or bending for at least the first week
- Skin sutures out POD 5; staples (if used) POD 10
- Limited sun exposure for 6 weeks (longer if they have had resurfacing)
- Review at 6 weeks (wounds), 3 months and final at 6 months
- Downtime before socially presentable (depends on adjuncts):
  - SMAS procedures 3–4 weeks
  - Periosteal procedures 6–8 weeks

Risks/Complications

Haematoma
Nerve injury
Wound healing problems, i.e., skin slough, infection
Fixation failure, i.e., pixie ear, altered hairline
Scarring

Outcome

Patients tend to be very pleased. Minor problems often settle. Wait at least 9 months before revisions/redos.

Terminology

Types of facelift
Composite – SMAS and skin kept as one layer (good for smokers)
Deep plane – sub SMAS plane
Biplanar – supra and sub-SMAS planes developed and may be moved in different vectors
Extended – SMAS dissection past zygomaticus major
SMASectomy – excision of part of SMAS

Volumetric – use of Coleman fat to add volume with minimal skin incisions

Minimal access techniques

MACS – Minimal Access Cranial Suspension lift; involves incision in front of and above the ear. Variation on S-lift and other short scar techniques

Threads – barbed suture to resuspend; no longer advocated

Key names

Mitz & Peyronie, Skoog – described SMAS
Baker/Stuzin – Extended SMAS lift
Krastinova – MASK lift
Bessin/Little/Ramirez – midface lifting
Hamra – composite/deep plane
Marten – MACS
Vasconez – endoscopic browlift

Chapter 24
Nerve Compression

Shehan Hettiaratchy, Abhilash Jain, and Jon Simmons

Think neck down but remember carpal and cubital tunnel are common, the rest rare.

Recognition

Female, middle aged. May have no obvious visible physical signs (Fig. 24.1).

History

General intro
Age, occupation, handedness, hobbies

Specific
When did it start?
Did anything trigger it off? Any previous history of neck/elbow/wrist trauma (may cause traction on the nerve, e.g., distal radius fracture or supracondylar humeral fracture, or nerve compression, e.g., degenerative foraminal stenosis in the neck).

S. Hettiaratchy (✉)
Department of Plastic and Reconstructive Surgery,
Imperial College Healthcare NHS Trust,
London, UK

S. Hettiaratchy et al. (eds.), *Plastic Surgery*,
DOI 10.1007/978-1-84882-116-3_24,
© Springer-Verlag London Limited 2012

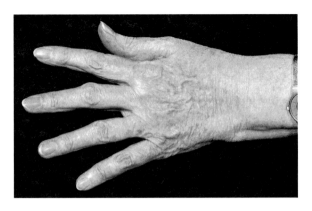

FIGURE 24.1 Wasting of first dorsal interosseous

Unilateral or bilateral – bilateral suggests neck might be the source
Specifically what symptoms do they get?

Type	Pins and needles/numbness/aching/pain/ burning
Radiation	Proximal – into neck?
	Distal – into fingers – which ones? Ask specifically about thumb/index and little
	Is the back of the hand affected? (dorsal branch ulnar nerve – differentiates between cubital tunnel and Guyon's canal entrapment)
	Is the palm affected? (palmar cutaneous branch median nerve – if it is affected then it is likely to be more proximal compression that carpal tunnel)
Timing	Nocturnal
	Diurnal – associated with more severe compression
Triggers	Wrist flexed (carpal tunnel) – holding phone/driving
	Pressure on medial elbow (cubital tunnel) – leaning on a desk

Motor	Clumsiness/dropping things – either due to weakness or proprioceptive impairment
	Weak grip – either median or ulnar nerve
	Weak wrist/finger extension – radial nerve (radial tunnel syndrome)
Interventions	Splinting at night (carpal tunnel)
	Steroid injections – did they work and for how long
Vascular	Only ask if there is a suggestion of TOCS; symptoms of ischaemia, especially positional
Activities	Affect on work and ADLs

Risk factors

Need to exclude causes of intrinsic nerve damage – DM, neuropathy (ask about other nerves such as feet/vision), neurotoxic drugs

Causes of compression – pregnancy, acromegaly, hypothyroid, systemic steroids

Predisposing factors – DM, relative ischaemia makes the nerve more vulnerable to compression

AIM: by the end of history you should

1. Know which nerves are likely to be affected
2. Know severity and duration
3. Know likelihood of reversibility/causative and contributing factors
4. Have considered likely level

Examination

Look

Signs of wasting:

| TOCS/plexopathy | check muscle groups of upper limb, especially biceps (C5,6) |

Median	Low – Thenar muscle wasting.
Ulnar	Low – Intrinsics (guttering between metacarpals)/ fist web due to adductor pollicis + first dorsal interosseous wasting.
Radial	Radial tunnel unlikely to give wasting; if there is forearm wasting think of lesion in spiral groove.

Feel/move
Sensory exam

Test	Thumb/index tip (Median)
	Palm (PCBMN – unaffected in carpal tunnel usually)
	Little finger (Ulnar)
	Dorsum ulnar half (DBUN – preserved in Guyon's, affected in cubital tunnel)
	First web (Radial)

Motor exam

Test	Wrist and finger extension (Radial)
	Wrist and finger flexion (Ulnar and Median)
	Opposition (Median)
	Finger adduction (Ulnar)
	Thumb adduction (Ulnar)
	Thumb flexion (Median via FPL)

Provocative tests

| Test | Test Tinel's on carpal/radial/cubital tunnels |
| | Phalen's test - Direct pressure on carpal tunnel/ Guyon's canal |

AIM: by the end of exam you should

1. Know which nerves are affected
2. Identify the level of compression
3. Formulate a management strategy

Treatment

Median nerve at wrist (Carpal tunnel)
Carpal tunnel release either open or endoscopic. Non-operative management for selected patients e.g.,). Mild symptoms in pregnancy may resolve post-partum.

Median nerve in forearm (Pronator syndrome)
Compression can be under Pronator Terres, FDS arch, Ligament of Struthers and bicipital aponeurosis. Treat with decompression.

Ulnar nerve at the wrist (Guyon's canal)
Release Guyon's canal through incision along radial border of FCU.

Ulnar nerve at the elbow (Cubital tunnel syndrome)
Simple decompression vs. medial epicondylectomy vs. anterior transposition in a subcutaneous or submuscular plane.

Radial nerve (Radial tunnel syndrome)
Surgical release using either an anterolateral or posterior approach

Outcome

Established motor weakness may not improve, aim to intervene before this point
1–3% nerve injury depending on procedure
5% delayed healing
<1% ischemia
Pillar pain

Anatomy

Median nerve
Compression at the wrist is in the carpal tunnel.
In the forearm may be under Pronator Terres, FDS arch, Ligament of Struthers or bicipital aponeurosis.

Ulna nerve

At the elbow compression is through the cubital tunnel, Arcade of Struthers, medial intermuscular septum and the 2 heads of FCU.

At the wrist through Guyon's canal.

Radial nerve

Compression through the radial tunnel may be from the leash of Henry, Arcade of Frohse or a fibrous band tethering the radial nerve to the radio-humoral joint.

Anterior Interosseous Nerve

Compression of purely motor branch of median nerve supplying FPL, Pronator Quadratus and FDP to index and middle. Compression is caused by an aberrant head of FPL (Ganzer's muscle), aberrant radial artery or fibrous band in Pronator Terres or FDS. Results in inability to form an 'O' between thumb and index.

Posterior Interosseous nerve

Compression of distal branch of radial nerve in the forearm results in preserved sensation in superficial radial nerve distribution but weakness in forearm extensors. Causes of compression are lipoma, tumour, RA involving radial head and trauma in the form of radial head fracture or elbow dislocation.

Papers

Skoff, Hillel D. M.D.; Sklar, Robin OTR/L CHT. Endoscopic Median Nerve Decompression: Early Experience. Plastic & Reconstructive Surgery. 94(5):691–694, October 1994.

Controversies

Endoscopic vs. open approach for carpal tunnel release
Cubital tunnel – simple release vs. epicondylectomy vs. anterior transposition
Simple decompression vs. neurolysis

Chapter 25
Severe Soft Tissue Infection

Jon Simmons, Shehan Hettiaratchy, and Carolyn Hemsley

Must identify infections requiring immediate operative treatment. Necrotising fasciitis is a surgical emergency and requires immediate operative treatment.

Recognition

The key question should be: is this necrotising fasciitis or severe cellulitis?

Necrotising fasciitis:	Rapidly progressing (less than 24 h)
	Very sick patient (septic, acidotic, coagulopathic)
	Patches of skin infarction with viable skin in between. Elevated Lactate.
Severe cellulitis:	Longer history (>24 h)
	Patient less sick (raised WCC but not septic/acidotic/coagulopathic)
	Skin red/blistering but not infracted

J. Simmons (✉)
Department of Plastic and Reconstructive Surgery,
Imperial College Healthcare NHS Trust,
London, UK

S. Hettiaratchy et al. (eds.), *Plastic Surgery*,
DOI 10.1007/978-1-84882-116-3_25,
© Springer-Verlag London Limited 2012

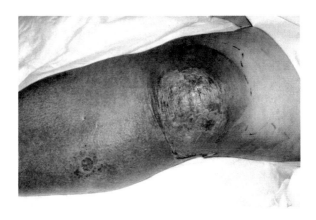

FIGURE 25.1 Cellulitis or necrotising fasciitis?

NB: Beware atypical infections, cellulitis refractory to antibiotics. If in doubt explore surgically and involve Microbiology
early (Fig. 25.1).

History

General intro
Age, occupation – particularly at risk of unusual organisms –
working with animals/outdoors/water
Health status prior to current illness

Specific
Rate of progression critical
Possible source of infection – minor wounds/injuries

Risk factors
IDDM
Immunoincompetence – immunosuppression/HIV
IVDU
Obesity
Age >60

PVD

NSAID

AIM: by the end of history you should know

1. Does the time course make a necrotising infection likely
2. Does the patient have a predisposing risk factor for infection
3. Are unusual organisms likely

Examination

Look

Does the patient look sick?

Are they shocked – hypotensive, peripherally shutdown, oligo/anuric?

Are they pyrexial?

What does the affected tissue look like?

Cellulitis – red, angry, tissues (especially with streptococcus – erysipelas)

Necrotising fasciitis – skin is dead; non-perfused, infarcted, necrotic, may smell dead/necrotic

Feel/move

Cellulitis may be hot and tender; necrotising fasciitis may be tender but may not be hot

Is there subcutaneous crepitus (37% of necrotising fasciitis has surgical emphysema)?

Move any suspicious joints – possibly septic arthritis

Any subcutaneous collections; cellulitis may result from deep seated infection/abscess

Needle test areas suspected of infarction if not clearly demarcated

AIM: by the end of exam

1. Determine if it is necrotising fasciitis or cellulitis
2. Find out how sick the patient is
3. Have a surgical plan – urgency/extent of surgery

Investigations

Imaging
Should not delay surgical management for imaging unless patient is well and diagnosis uncertain/atypical. XR – 57% necrotising fasciitis shows air in the soft tissues. Ultrasound (good to demonstrate collections), CT, MRI if diagnosis unclear.

Bloods
Baseline FBC (WCC, Hb and neutrophils), clotting (DIC, coagulopathic), U + E (Renal impairment), lactate and arterial blood gases, inflammatory markers and blood cultures.

Microbiology
Microbiology – get samples before antibiotics. Swab any open wounds. Any obvious pus send off. Aspirate and send off any blister fluid – put some in a blood cultures bottle. Take 2 sets of blood cultures. FNA swab aspirate may be useful in cellulitis.

Beware – severe cellulitis can make the patient very sick with sepsis etc. but the clinical and blood picture tend not to be as deranged as necrotising fasciitis, especially degree of acidosis.

Treatment

Severe cellulitis requires aggressive non-surgical management. Necrotising fasciitis requires aggressive surgical management.

Cellulitis
Resuscitation of the patient as can be shocked
High dose antibiotics – empirical initially then directed
Strict elevation of any affected limb
If it involves the hand then splintage in James position (position of safety) is needed

If there is any suggestion of a subcutaneous collection this must be drained. USS may be useful to confirm a collection.

If there is any doubt about the diagnosis then surgery with an exploration of the tissues and fascial biopsy may be helpful.

Necrotising fasciitis
This is a surgical emergency, resuscitate the patient and correct coagulopathy.

Surgery – aggressive debridement of all suspicious tissue. Cut 1–2 cm into viable tissue to confirm clear margins. Multiple specimens for micro (tissue and fluid) and histology – send all urgently for gram stain and culture.

IV antibiotics – broad spectrum (local micro policy) and then focussed based on cultures. Example: Ceftriaxone + clindamycin + gentamicin

Return to theatre within 24 h to check for progression/viability of debrided tissue

Patient will need SSG once they no longer have overt infection and then may require delayed recon after to improve aesthetics/function.

Outcome

Mortality for necrotising fasciitis is 6–71%.

Pearls

Micro:
Classified by what grows
Type 1 – Polymicrobial; trauma, surgery with risk factors. May look like cellulitis
Type 2 – Group A streptococcus+/– anaerobe; ?NSAID; trauma, surgery, IVDU, childbirth
Type 3 – Clostridial – myonecrosis

Coined by Wilson 1962
Mortality 6–71%
Due to toxin production

Group A strep: M type 1–3 – M = surface protein that prevents phagocytosis and increases adherence + exotoxin produces an inflammatory process which progresses along fascial planes and causes infraction of skin perforators and hence skin infarction.

Clindamycin decreases exotoxin production, hence is often used in conjunction with other bacteriocidal antibiotics.

Key Evidences

Kotrappa KS, Bansal RS, Amin NM. Necrotizing fasciitis. Am Fam Phys 1996;53(5):1691–6.

Forbes N, Rankin APN. Necrotizing fasciitis and nonsteroidal antiinflammatory drugs: A case series and review of the literature. N Z Med J 2001;114:3–6.

Urschel JD. Necrotizing soft tissue infections. Postgrad Med J 1999;75:645–9. (Excellent review article)

Controversies

Hyperbaric oxygen treatment
If a diagnosis of necrotising fasciitis is obvious, likely or possible surgical exploration must be undertaken as an emergency. Beware the 'cellulitis' patient deteriorating on broad spectrum antibiotic treatment who is becoming increasingly unwell.

Chapter 26
Rhinoplasty

John Henton and Jon Simmons

Refers to open or closed procedures to alter the size or shape of the nose. It is performed for aesthetic, functional or reconstructive indications. Beware the man who 'just doesn't like' his nose.

Recognition

Cosmesis is the most common reason for performing rhinoplasty. Patients may feel their nose is too crooked, large or protruding. It may be deformed following trauma, or excision of malignancy. The deformity may also be secondary to congenital defects or scar contracture following cleft lip correction as a child. There may be functional impairment, with the patient complaining of difficulty breathing through one or both nostrils. Over 4,000 rhinoplasty procedures were carried out in the UK by BAAPS members in 2010 (Fig. 26.1).

J. Henton (✉)
Department of Plastic and Reconstructive Surgery,
Imperial College Healthcare NHS Trust,
London, UK

S. Hettiaratchy et al. (eds.), *Plastic Surgery*,
DOI 10.1007/978-1-84882-116-3_26,
© Springer-Verlag London Limited 2012

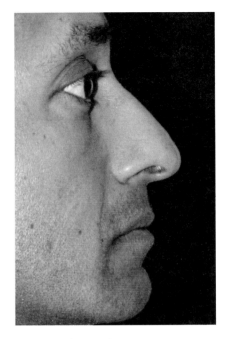

FIGURE 26.1 Pre-operative patient

Anatomy

Soft tissue cover

- Skin – thinner, less sebaceous upper 2/3, thicker more sebaceous lower 1/3
- Musculoaponeurotic layer

Structural support
Bony/cartilaginous skeleton

- Upper 1/3 – nasal bones, ascending process of maxilla
- Middle 1/3 – upper lateral cartilages, dorsal cartilaginous septum
- Lower 1/3 – lower lateral (alar) cartilages – lateral, medial and middle crus

Septum – Quadrangular cartilage, vomer, perpendicular plate of ethmoid, nasal spine

Blood supply

- Angular artery, superior labial artery, columellar artery (branches of facial artery)
- Arterial supply runs in submusculoaponeurotic plane (superior to perichondrium)
- Venous/lymphatics – subcutaneous plane
- Sensation – Via V1 and V2 branches of trigeminal nerve

Lining – Squamous epithelium in vestibule, changing to ciliated columnar respiratory epithelium.

The nasal aesthetic subunits; dorsum, lobule, sidewalls, alae, columella, soft triangles.

History

General introduction

Age, occupation (do they rely on their sense of smell for work: chef, wine taster etc.). Reasons for seeking rhinoplasty, interference with: lifestyle, relationships, self-confidence.

Nose specific

- What EXACTLY do they not like about their nose?
  - Is the procedure for aesthetic, functional (or a combination of both) reasons?
  - Their expectations from rhinoplasty surgery
  - Beware patients who cannot specifically point out which features of their nose they do not like (?body dysmorphic disorder)
- Any previous nasal surgery?
- Facial/nasal trauma
- Breathing difficulties
- Sense of smell (can be damaged during surgery)
- Epistaxis
- Allergic rhinitis
- Use of nasal decongestants
- Cocaine use – risk of septal necrosis/perforation/poor results (Slavin PRS 1990)
- Awareness of risks and complications associated with surgery

Risk factors

- Few absolute contraindications
- Significant past medical history of cardiac, GI or respiratory problems (this can potentially interfere with post-op recovery/mobilisation and increase risk of complications)
- Smoking (despite excellent blood supply to nose)
- Anticoagulants
- Bleeding tendencies

General

Full medical and drug history.

- Must consider co-existing morbidities relative to risks of procedure (usually a purely cosmetic procedure)
- Autoimmune conditions – e.g., Wegner's, sarcoid (can cause saddle nose due to septum collapse)
- Full list of medications such as aspirin, NSAIDs, herbal medications, anticoagulants
- Any psychological issues (i.e., is patient requesting surgery for genuine reasons)
- Occupation and sporting hobbies (as this may interfere with these)
- Any drug allergies
- Smoking

AIM: by the end of history you should

1. Know the patient's motivation for rhinoplasty
2. Understand exactly what they hope to achieve from surgery
3. Be aware any co-morbidities which will impact on the procedure/post-op recovery
4. Know of the need for additional investigations/treatment of any co-morbidities prior to surgery
5. Have identified if the patient is seeking surgery for appropriate reasons (identify patient with body dismorphic disorder)

Examination

Look
Whole face

- Divide face into thirds to assess proportions
- Is it really their nose which is an abnormal shape/size – or other facial features

Nose
Sit opposite patient and at same level. View from front:

- Nose should occupy middle vertical 1/3 of face
- Width (alar base width) should be same as intercanthal distance
- Look for asymmetry or deviation of dorsum
- Assess skin quality and thickness
    - Thin skin shows alterations to bony/cartilaginous framework much more obviously than thick skin. Skin drapes better, but minor imperfections more obvious.
    - If skin thick and sebaceous, need to make much more dramatic alterations to framework to achieve a visible effect.

View from side

- Radix should be at same level as upper lid eyelashes
- Tip projection – should be same as alar base width
- Nasofrontal angle
- Nasolabial angle – 95–100 degrees in females, 90–95 degrees for men
- Assess dorsum – straight? dorsal hump?
- Supratip/tip deformity
- Columellar show

View nasal base

- Should make equilateral triangle
- Assess septal deviation

Feel/move/measure
Cottle test – for internal nasal valve collapse
In a positive test; lateral traction on cheek opens valve improving airflow

- Indication for spreader graft.

AIM: by the end of exam you should

1. Have identified any previous unknown pathology which may require investigation/treatment
2. Understand the problem areas patient wishes to address
3. Have decided on most appropriate technique/combination of techniques
4. Awareness of patient's expectations of outcome

Investigations

- ENT for nasoendoscopy + biopsies if any history of cocaine use/suspicion of intranasal ca
- Routine bloods: FBC, U + Es, Coag
- May also need chest X-ray, ECG etc. depending on co-morbidities

Clinical Photography

- Anterior, lateral, oblique and basal views
- Important to document pre-operative appearance, both for planning surgery, any revisions and for medico-legal reasons

Treatment/Surgical Technique

Preparation
GA, shave nasal hairs with small blade, prep with chlorhexidine
Mark incision (step or chevron for columella)
LA + Epinephrine infiltration
Topical vasoconstrictor nasal packs

Access: Open or closed approach
Open:

- Incision through narrowest part of columella
- Dissection continues in submusculoaponeurotic plane to avoid vascular damage

Closed:

- Intranasal incisions to access desired area

Intranasal incisions
Transcartilaginous: Incision through the structure of the lower lateral cartilage
Intracartilaginous: Incision placed between the caudal end of the upper lateral and the cephalic margin of the lower lateral cartilage
Marginal: Incision courses along the caudal margin of the lower lateral cartilage

Augmentation/reduction manoeuvres
Tip reshaping with sutures
Onlay graft – Improve tip projection
Umbrella graft – Augments septal tip support
Dorsal hump reduction
Dorsal graft – to raise/support dorsum – e.g., to correct saddle deformity
Spreader grafts – Holds internal nasal valve open, widens nasal dorsum
Infracturing – Osteotomy to narrow nose or correct open roof deformity
Open roof deformity – Flattened appearance of dorsum following dorsal hump reduction

Risks/Complications

General

- DVT/PE/Chest infection

Specific to the nose
- Infection
- Haematoma
- Scarring (columella, open approach)
- Oedema
- Damage to nasal septum
- Altered sensation to nose/upper teeth
- Olfactory changes

Post-operative Management

- Home in evening or next day
- Analgesia, antibiotics +/– steroids
- Avoid any strenuous activity, heavy lifting, sports for minimum of 4 weeks
- Downtime: can be back at sedentary occupation after 2 weeks
- Sutures out at 5 days
- Splint off at 1 week
- Counsel about: duration of oedema – 3 months

Controversies: Open Versus Closed Rhinoplasty

Open rhinoplasty
- Advantages
  - Better visualisation of osteocartilagenous skeleton
  - Better access to nasal cartilages for grafts
  - Able to make more dramatic alterations to dorsum, tip etc
  - Direct access to tissues for haemostasis
- Disadvantages
  - Scar across columella
  - Delayed healing/prolonged recovery
  - Longer duration of swelling

Closed Rhinoplasty

- Advantages
  - No external scarring
  - Vascular bridges preserved
  - Faster recovery

- Less post-op swelling
- Allows creation of pockets into which grafts can be placed
- Disadvantages
  - Poor visualisation of operative field
  - Difficult dissection

Appendix: FRCS Plast Classification Systems

Contents

- Aesthetic
- Cancer Staging
- Craniofacial
- Congenital
- General
- Hand
- Reconstruction/Flaps
- Trauma
- Incidences
- Other Useful Bits for the Exam

Aesthetic

Baker, Capsule Formation 1975

I – No capsule
II – Palpable
III – Visible
IV – Painful

Heimburg, Tuberous breast, *BJPS*, 1996;49:339–345

Type 1: Hypoplasia of infero-medial quadrant
Type 2: Hypoplasia of both inferior quadrants
Type 3: Hypoplasia of both lower quadrants and subareolar skin shortage
Type 4: Severely constricted base

Matarasso Classification of Abdominoplasty

Type 1: Excess fat only – liposuction
Type 2: Mild skin excess, infra-umbilical divarification – mini-abdominoplasty infra-umbilical plication liposuction

S. Hettiaratchy et al. (eds.), *Plastic Surgery*,
DOI 10.1007/978-1-84882-116-3,
© Springer-Verlag London Limited 2012

Type 3: Moderate skin excess, infra and superior divarification – As above

Type 4: Severe skin excess – Standard abdominoplasty with plication and liposuction

Paysk zones around an expander

Inner zone:	Fibrin layer with macrophages
Central zone:	Fibroblasts and myofibroblasts
Transitional zone:	Loose collagen
Outer zone:	Blood vessels and collagen

Regnault classification of ptosis

1st degree: Nipples at or above IMF

2nd degree: Nipples below IMF but above most dependant portion of the breast

3rd degree: Nipples below the most dependant portion of the breast

• Pseudo-ptosis – where the majority of the breast mound lies below the IMF but nipple is above or on the IMF. Post BBR common

Simon classification for gynaecomastia

Stage 1:   Slight volume increase no excess skin

Stage 2a: Moderate volume increase without excess skin

Stage 2b: Moderate volume increase with excess skin

Stage 3:   Marked volume increase with excess skin

Cancer Staging

Broder's histological grading of SCC

Grade I:	Well differentiated Ratio Diff:Undiff	3:1
Grade II:	Mod differentiated Ratio Diff:Undiff	1:1
Grade III:	Poorly differentiated Ratio	1:3
Grade IV:	Undifferentiated	

TNM classification for cutaneous melanoma

Classification	Thickness (mm)	Ulceration status/Mitoses
T		
Tis	NA	NA
T1	≤1.00	a: Without ulceration and mitosis < $1/mm^2$
		b: With ulceration or mitoses ≥ $1/mm^2$
T2	1.01–2.00	a: Without ulceration
		b: With ulceration
T3	2.01–4.00	a: Without ulceration
		b: With ulceration
T4	>4.00	a: Without ulceration
		b: With ulceration
N	*No. of metastatic nodes*	*Nodal metastatic burden*
N0	0	NA
N1	1	a: Micrometastasis[*]
		b: Macrometastasis[†]
N2	2–3	a: Micrometastasis[*]
		b: Macrometastasis[†]
		c: In-transit metastases/satellites without metastatic nodes
N3	4+	metastatic nodes, or matted nodes, or in-transit metastases/satellites with metastatic nodes
M	*Site*	*Serum LDH*
M0	No distant metastases	NA
M1a	Distant skin, subcutaneous, or nodal metastases	Normal
M1b	Lung metastases	Normal
M1c	All other visceral metastases	Normal
	Any distant metastasis	Elevated

AJCC classification 2009

	Clinical staging				Pathologic staging		
	T	N	M		T	N	M
0	Tis	N0	M0	0	Tis	N0	M0
IA	T1a	N0	M0	IA	T1a	N0	M0
IB	T1b	N0	M0	IB	T1b	N0	M0
	T2a	N0	M0		T2a	N0	M0
IIA	T2b	N0	M0	IIA	T2b	N0	M0
	T3a	N0	M0		T3a	N0	M0
IIB	T3b	N0	M0	IIB	T3b	N0	M0
	T4a	N0	M0		T4a	N0	M0
IIC	T4b	N0	M0	IIC	T4b	N0	M0
III	Any T	N > N0	M0	IIIA	T1-4a	N1a	M0
					T1-4a	N2a	M0
				IIIB	T1-4b	N1a	M0
					T1-4b	N2a	M0
					T1-4a	N1b	M0
					T1-4a	N2b	M0
					T1-4a	N2c	M0
				IIIC	T1-4b	N1b	M0
					T1-4b	N2b	M0
					T1-4b	N2c	M0
					Any T	N3	M0
IV	Any T	Any N	M1	IV	Any T	Any N	M1

Enneking sarcoma staging

Stage	Grade	Anatomical location	Metastasis
0	Benign (G0)	Any	None
IA	Low (G1)	Intra-compartmental (T1)	None
IB	Low	Extra-compartmental (T2)	None
IIA	High (G2)	Intra-compartmental	None
IIB	High	Extra-compartmental	None
III	Any	Any	Mets (M1)

AJCC for sarcoma

Stage	Grade	Size (cm)	Metastasis	Relationship to fascia
IA	Low	<5	None	Any
IB	Low	>5	None	Superficial
IIA	Low	>5	None	Deep
IIB	High	<5	None	Any
IIC	High	>5	None	Superficial
III	High	>5	None	Deep
IV	Any	Any	Yes	Any

Trojani histological grading system: sarcoma

- Basis of this grading system is based on the following
  - Histology
  - Mitosis
  - Necrosis
  - Differentiation
  - Stroma
  - Number of cells

Tumours of the head and neck

	Oral cavity (cm)	Nasopharynx	Hypopharynx	Maxillary sinus
T1	<2	1 subsite	1 subsite	Mucosal only
T2	2–4	>1 subsite	>1 subsite not fixed	Into bone below Ohngrens line[a]
T3	>4	Beyond nasal cavity	Into larynx	Into bone above Ohngrens line[a]
T4	Invades adjacent structures	Skull base or CN	Into neck soft tissues	Invades adjacent structures

[a]Medial canthus to angle of the mandible
For salivary gland tumours add A or B to the T stage to
signify no local extension or local extension
Nodal classification:

N1:   Single ipsilateral <3 cm
N2a: Single ipsilateral 3–6 cm
N2b: Multiple ipsilateral not >6 cm
N2c: Bilateral or contralateral nodes 3–6 cm
N3:   Any node >6 cm

TNM staging for head and neck cancer

Stage 1	T1	N0	M0
Stage 2	T2	N0	M0
Stage 3	T3	N0	M0
	<T4	N1	M0
Stage 4	T4	N0	M0
	Any T	N2/3	M0
	Any T	Any N	M1

Classification of neck dissection

- Comprehensive
  - Radical
    - 5 levels
    - IJV, AN, SCM
  - Modified radical (functional)
    - T1 – preserves the AN
    - T2 – preserves the AN and SCM
    - T3 – preserves AN, SCM and IJV
  - Extended radical
    - May take parotid, mediastinal nodes or paratracheal nodes

- Selective neck dissection
  - Supraomohyoid
    - Oral cavity tumours
    - Levels 1,2 and 3
  - Anterolateral
    - Laryngeal and hypopharynx tumours
    - Levels 2,3 and 4
  - Anterior
    - Thyroid tumours
    - Levels 2,3 and 4 with tracheo-oesophageal nodes
  - Posterior
    - Posterior scalp
    - Levels 2,3,4 and 5

WHO classification of salivary gland tumours

1. Adenoma
   (a) Pleomorphic
   (b) Warthin's – Adenolymphoma
   (c) Oncocytoma

2. Carcinoma
   (a) Muco-epidermoid
       (i) Well, inter and poorly differentiated grades. Well and inter OK
   (b) Malignant mixed tumour – arising in PMA
   (c) Acinic cell
   (d) Adenocarcinoma
   (e) Adenoid cystic – Szanto's grades
       (i) Grade 1 – cibrose, no solidity good prognosis
       (ii) Grade 2 – tubular, <30% solid
       (iii) Grade 3 – solid, poor prognosis
   (f) Squamous cell
3. Non-epithelial tumours
4. Malignant lymphomas
5. Secondary tumours
   (a) MM
   (b) SCC
   (c) Breast
   (d) Thyroid
6. Unclassified
7. Tumour like
   (a) Oncocytosis
   (b) Sialadenosis
   (c) Cysts
   (d) Infection
   (e) Granulomatous disease

Craniofacial

Knight and North classification of malar fractures 1961

Type 1:   Undisplaced fractures
Type 2:   *Isolated # of the arch – STABLE AFTER REDUCTION*
Type 3:   Unrotated body fracture
Type 4:   Medially rotated # of the body
Type 5:   *Laterally rotated # of the body – STABLE AFTER REDUCTION*
Type 6:   Complex

Manson classification of malar fractures – based on CT findings

Type 1:   *Low energy* fractures – result in little or no displacement. Often ZF#

Type 2:   *Medium energy* – # of all buttresses, mod displacement, comminution

Often require intra-oral and eyelid incisions to fix

Type 3:   *High energy* – Frequently occur with Le Fort or panfacial #. Posterior dislocation of arch and malar eminence. Requires coronal, eyelid and intra-oral incisions

Angle classification of dental occlusion

• Occlusion defined as the relative position of the upper first molar. Mesiobuccal cusp should rest in mesiobuccal groove of mandibular first molar

Class 1:   Normal occlusion but other problems e.g., overcrowding

Class 2:   Overbite, retrognathism

Class 3:   Underbite, prognathism, negative overjet

Le Fort classification of maxillary fractures

LeFort I: Tooth bearing maxilla separated from midface. Fracture through pterygoid

Plates to piriform aperture through maxilla

LeFort II: Pyramidal fracture

Extends from frontonasal junction along medial orbital wall, IO Rim and posteriorly through pterygoid plates

LeFort III: Craniofacial dysjunction .# Extends out through the lateral orbital wall through the zygoma and high through the pterygoid plates

Classification of craniofacial anomalies – American Society of Cleft Lip/Palate

1. Clefts
2. Synostosis
   (a)   Syndromal
   (b)   Non-syndromal
3. Hypoplastic conditions
   (a)   TC
   (b)   Hemifacial microsomia – OMENS classification
   (c)   Hemifacial atrophy – Rombergs

4. Hyperplastic conditions
   Fibrous dysplasia – abnormal proliferation of bone form-
   ing mesenchyme, maxillary/mandibular mass, osseous
   lesions, Albrights including precocious puberty, cafe au
   lait, pituitary tumours

Tessier's classification for hyperteliorism

Type 1: IOD 30–34 mm
Type 2: IOD 35–39 mm
Type 3: IOD 40 mm+

Veau's classification 1931

1. Incomplete cleft of secondary palate
2. Complete cleft of secondary palate
3. Complete unilateral cleft lip and palate
4. Bilateral cleft lip and palate

Striped Y classification

1. First described by Kernahan and Stark 1958
2. Modified by Millard and Seider 1977
3. Pictorial classification

Craniofacial syndromes
Aperts – 1:160,000

- Bicoronal synostosis – turricephaly/brachycephaly
- Midface hypoplasia
- Beaked nose
- Class 3 occlusion
- CP 20%
- **Complex syndactyly**
  - T1 – Thumb and little finger separate
  - T2 – Thumb separate
  - T3 – Involves all the hand

Crouzon – 1:15,000 AD

- Bicoronal synostosis – turricephaly/brachycephaly
- Midface hypoplasia
- Exorbitism
- **Normal hands**

Saethre-Chotzen

- Bicoronal synostosis
- Low hair line
- Ptosis
- Small posterior ears
- **Simple syndactyly**

Pfeiffer

- Similar appearance to Aperts
- **Broad thumbs and toes**

Carpenter syndrome – rare

- Various sutures involved
- **Pre-axial polydactyly**
- **Partial syndactyly**

Treacher-Collins syndrome

- Chromosome 5 TCOF gene coding for Treacle protein
- AD 1:15,000
- Bilateral features
- Beaked narrowed nose
- Micrognathia
- Confluent 6,7,8 cleft
- Colomboma
- Medial lashes absent
- Malar hypoplasia
- Microtia
- CP

Romberg's hemifacial atrophy

- Acquired condition
- Usually unilateral
- Sporadic
- Usually starts aged between 5 and late teens
- Do nothing while disease is active
- Results in permanent soft tissue atrophy
  - Skin
  - Hair

- Iris
- Forehead
- Cheek
- Skeleton

Goldenhars – OMENS+ classification

- 1 in 5,000
- 90% unilateral
- Ocular, mandibular, ear, facial nerve and normally sporadic
- Goldenhar's consists of hemifacial microsomia, vertebral abnormalities and epibulbar dermoids

Prosanski classification of mandibular deformities in HFM/ Goldenhar's

Group 1: Mild mandibular hypoplasia
Group 2a: Severe hypoplasia with articulating TMJ
Group 2b: Severe without non-articulating TMJ
Group 3: Hypoplasia of mandibular ramus without a TMJ

Craniofacial clefts – Tessier

- Sporadic 1 in 25,000
- Aetiology unclear
    - Failure of fusion
    - Lack of mesoderm penetration
    - Amniotic bands

May occupy any or all layers of the face
Soft tissue defect does not necessarily correspond with the bony defect
Often have hairline markers
Facial clefts 1–7 (7 most lateral – corner of the mouth)
Cranial clefts 8–14 (8 most lateral – corner of the orbit)

0	Medial craniofacial dysraphia
	Associated with encephaloceles and hypertelorism
1	Between incisors then through nasal bone and frontal process of maxilla
	Bifid dome hypertelorism and wide bridge
2	Paranasal
	As for cleft 1

3	Oculonasal cleft
	Runs through nasal and lacrimal bones into the maxilla
	Medial orbit and lacrimal apparatus may be deficient
	Coloboma
	Lower portion passes through the lateral incisor and canine
4	Oculofacial 1 cleft
	More lateral to 3 medial to the IOF
5	Oculofacial 2 cleft
	Lateral to IOF
	Central coloboma
6	Between maxilla and zygoma
	Lateral lower lid coloboma
	TC with 7 and 8
7	Between zygoma and temporal bone
	May extend medially to the corner of the mouth across the cheek
8	Outwards from the lateral canthus
9,10,11	Start in supraorbital region associated with 3,4 and 5
12,13,14	Do not involve the orbit
	Extensions of 0,1 and 2
30	Median cleft of lower lip and mandible
	May extend onto the neck

Congenital

Hand

Swanson classification of upper limb developmental anomalies
Failure of formation
   Transverse
   Longitudinal – radial, central, intercalated
Failure of differentiation
   Soft tissue – syndactyly
   Skeletal – Clinodactyly
Duplication
   Pre-axial
   Post-axial
   Central

Undergrowth
Overgrowth
Amniotic band syndrome/constriction ring syndrome
Generalised conditions
    Achondroplasia

Bayne and Klug classification for deficiencies of radius – 1987

- *Usually associated with a Blauth 4 or 5; exception is TAR*
- *Sporadic, syndromic (VATER, TAR, Cardiac, Fanconi's, Holt-Oram)*
- *Type 4 is most common > Type 1 > Type 3 > Type 2 (Rare)*
- *½ bilateral*
- *1 in 50,000 (2 times more common than ulna dysplasia)*
- *R > L (Opposite to ulna dysplasia)*
- *M > F (M=F in UD)*
- *If managed surgically manage radius at 6–9/12 and thumb at 9–18/12*

Type 1:   Short distal radius – do nothing
Type 2:   Hypoplastic radius – can lengthen
Type 3:   Partial absence – centralisation
Type 4:   Complete absence – centralisation

Ulna dysplasia classification – Bayne

- *Use 1 classification for forearm and another for the hand*
- *BAYNE for forearm and Cole and Manske for the thumb and first web*
- *Associated with other musculoskeletal anomalies, scoliosis, hemimelia not systemic probs*
- *Reconstruct thumb, correct web space deformity, align wrist and forearm, stabilise wrist*
- *Rebalance wrist with tendon transfers*
- *Usually have good function*

Type 1:   Hypoplastic ulna
Type 2:   Partially absent ulna
Type 3:   Absent ulna
Type 4:   Humeroradial synostosis

Ulna dysplasia classification – Cole and Manske

- *Based on the thumb and first web*
- *70% have thumb anomaly*
- *30% have syndactyly*

Type A: Normal

Type B: Mild first web and thumb deficiency (Narrow)

Type C: Moderate to severe deformity with thumb/index
         syndactyly, lack of opposition thumb in palmar plane,
         thumb hypoplasia, lack of thumb extensors

Type D: Absent thumb

Upton classification of camptodactyly

- *Theories: Abnormal lumbrical insertion, extra or abnormal*
  FDS slips, abnormal extensor or PIPJ capsular structures

Type 1:   Congenital, isolated usually D5 M=F

Type 2:   Like type 1 but becomes clinically evident 7–11 years

Type 3:   Severe, congenital multiple digits associated with

          Trisomy 13–15, short stature syndromes, craniofacial
          syndromes

          Arthrogryposis

Symbrachydactyly types

Peromelic	nubbins
Short finger	type telescoping fingers
Cleft hand type	ulnar side cleft
Monodactylous	single digit

Typical cleft versus atypical cleft (symbrachydactyly) hand

Typical	Atypical
Bilateral	Unilateral
Feet involved	Feet spared
Starts on radial side	Starts on ulnar side
Little finger preserved	Thumb preserved
+ve Family history	–ve Family history

Adams classification of camptodactyly

Type 1:   Flexion contracture of PIPJ

Type 2:   Partially fixed

Type 3:   Arthrographically fixed

          3A – No x-ray changes

          3B – With x-ray changes – Wedged shaped (Anvil) P1 head, divot in the base of P2, subcondylar recess (Drucker's space), PIPJ slopes to ulna side

Type 4:   More than one digit involved

Stelling classification for polydactyly

- Ulna polydactyly very common 1:300 African Americans 1:3,000 Caucasians

Type 1:   No skeletal tissue

Type 2:   Skeletal attachment to enlarged or bifid phalynx/metacarpal

Type 3:   Complete duplication including a metacarpal

Tetamy classification for polydactyly

Preaxial

Type 1: Bony duplication (Wassel 1–6)
Type 2: Triphalangia
Type 3: Duplication of index finger
Type 4: Synpolydactyly (Syndactyly of D3/D4 fingers + toes +/– polydactyly of same)

Postaxial

Type 1: Fully developed extra ray
Type 2: Rudimentary extra ray

Wassel classification for thumb duplication

- *Bilhaut-Cloquet procedure for 1–3*
- *4–6 Preserve UCL, ID and preserve Abd PB, shell out radial thumb, k-wire for 4 weeks*

Type 1:   Duplicated distal phalynx (BIFID) – least common

Type 2:   Duplicated IPJ

Type 3:   Duplicated proximal phalynx

Type 4:   Duplicated MCPJ – most common

Type 5:   Duplicated metacarpal

Type 6: Duplicated CMCJ
Type 7: Tri-phalangia

Blauth classification of thumb hypoplasia

- *Types 3B, 4 and 5 best managed with pollicisation; 1-3A reconstruction of soft tissues*

Type 1: Minor hypoplasia
Type 2: Adduction contracture, thenar hypoplasia, normal skeleton
Type 3: Significant hypoplasia, skeletal hypoplasia, intrinsic muscle hypoplasia
         Rudimentary extrinsic tendons
         3A: CMCJ OK
         3B: CMCJ absent
Type 4: Floating thumb
Type 5: Absence

Weckesser clasp thumb

Type 1: Deficient thumb extension
Type 2: Deficient extension with flexion contracture
Type 3: Thumb hypoplasia
Type 4: Pre-axial polydactyly with deficient extension

Upton classification of macrodactyly

- *Index > middle > ring > thumb > little = very very rare*

Type 1: Macrodactyly associated with lipofibromatosis of nerve – median common
Type 2: Associated with NF1
Type 3: Macrodactyly with hyperostosis
Type 4: Macrodactyly with hemi-hypertrophy

Clinodactyly (Cooney)

Simple : bone <45°
Simple/complicated: bone >45°
Complex: soft tissue + bone <45° assoc. with syndactyly
Complex/complicated: soft tissue + bone>45°

Patterson classification: congenital constriction ring syndrome

- *Intrinsic theory – Internal defect in the embryo causing abnormalities*
- *Extrinsic theory – Amniotic band compresses or constricts extremity*

Type 1: Band with no distal deficit
Type 2: Band with distal lymphoedema
Type 3: Band with distal acrosyndactyly
Type 4: Distal auto-amputation

Vascular
Schobinger classification of arteriovenous malformations
Stage 1: Blue skin-blush
Stage 2: Mass assoc with bruit and thrill
Stage 3: Mass with ulceration, bleeding and pain
Stage 4: Stage 3 lesion producing heart failure

Waner grading system for capillary malformations

1. Sparce, pale non-confluent
2. Pink non-confluent
3. Discrete ectatic vessels
4. Confluent patch
5. Nodular lesion

Classification of vascular lesions (Mulliken and Glowacki, 82 *PRS*)

- *Haemangioma and vascular malformations in infants and children: a classification based on endothelial characteristics*
- Haemangioma and Vascular Malformations (high and low flow)

1.   Haemangioma
2a. Venous malformation
2b. Arterial malformation
2c. AV malformation
2d   Capillary malformation
2e. Lymphatic malformation

Enjolras and Mulliken, 2002 – New Classification

* Vascular tumours vs. vascular malformations

Classification of vascular lesions (Jackson et al., 1993)

Group I   Haemangioma
Group II   Vascular malformations
             A. Low flow – venous
             B. High flow – arteriovenous
Group III   Lymphatic malformations – lymphatico-venous

Other
Classification of hypospadius

1. Glanular
2. Coronal
3. Subcoronal
4. Distal shaft
5. Mid shaft
6. Proximal shaft
7. Penoscrotal
8. Scrotal
9. Perineal
   * Glanular, coronal and subcoronal termed distal and account for 85%

General

ASA grading of anaesthetic patients

ASA 1:   Normal healthy patient
ASA 2:   Patient with moderate systemic disease, or minor disease with operative or anaesthetic risks
ASA 3:   Patient with severe systemic disease limiting activity
ASA 4:   Severe incapacitating disease, constant threat to life
ASA 5:   Moribund, not expected to survive 24 h

Brachial plexus – Mellesi classification

1 – Supraganglionic
2 – Infraganglionic

3 – Trunk

4 – Cord

Fitzpatrick classification (Photosensitivity) (1988; *Arch Dermatol,* 124, 869–71)

Type 1:   Pale, white skin, red hair – always burns never tans

Type 2:   Fair skin blue eyes – burns easily tans poorly

Type 3:   Darker but white – tans after initial burn

Type 4:   Light brown skin – burns minimally, tans easily

Type 5:   Brown skin – rarely burns, tans darkly

Type 6:   Black or very dark – never burns, always dark tanning

House and Brackman grading of facial palsy

Measurement: Superior movement of mid-upper brow and lateral movement of the oral commissure. 1 point for each 2.5 mm up to a maximum of 10 mm. Points are then added

Grade 1:   8/8

Normal

Grade 2:   7/8

Slight weakness

At rest: normal tone and symmetry

Motion: Asymmetry of mouth, complete eye closure

Grade 3:   5–6/8

Obvious facial asymmetry, spasm

At rest: normal tone and symmetry

Motion: complete eye closure with effort, mouth weakness

Grade 4:   3–4/8

Disfiguring facial asymmetry with obvious weakness

No forehead movement

Incomplete eye closure

Grade 5:   1–2/8

Only slight movement

Grade 6:   No facial function

Lymphoedema

Primary lymphoedema

Lymphoedema congenital: Milroy's disease, 10–15% cases, abnormal lymphatic development. Familial. LL 3:1 UL. 2/3 both extremities

Hypoplasia or aplasia of SC lymphatics

Lymphoedema praecox:	65–80%. 70% due to segmental hypoplasia, other causes are aplasia and hyperplastic varicose lymphatics. Usually incompetent valves lead to lymphoedema. Presents at puberty Female 4:1 Male. Usually foot and ankle, 70% unilateral
Lymphoedema tarda:	Presents after 35 years. Possibly a spectrum of praecox where inadequate drainage to meet demands
Secondary lymphoedema:	Commonest cause CLND. Filariasis infection, TB, neoplasm and trauma

MRC classifications of nerve recovery

M0 – No contraction

M1 – Flicker

M2 – Muscle contraction with active motion with gravity eliminated

M3 – Full range of motion against gravity

M4 – Full range of motion against gravity with some resistance

M5 – Full range of motion against gravity with maximum resistance of that muscle

S0 – No sensibility

S1 – Recovery of deep cutaneous pain

S2 – Return of some superficial cutaneous pain and tactile sensibility

S3 – 2 point discrimination > 15mm

S3+ – 2 point discrimination 7–15mm

S4 – Normal. 2 point discrimination 3–6mm

Nerve injuries (Seddon 1948)

Neuropraxia	Loss of conduction
Axonotemesis	Loss of axon continuity may include endo-/perineurium
Neurotemesis	Complete severance

Nerve injuries (Sunderland 1968)

I	Loss of conduction
II	Loss of axonal continuity: axon only
III	Loss of axonal continuity: axon and endoneurium

IV   Loss of axonal continuity: axon, endoneurium and perineurium

V   Loss of axonal continuity: axon, endo-, peri- and epineurium

- Recovery – complete recovery should be observed with Sunderland I and II i.e. neuropraxia and axonotemesis

Pairolero and Arnold classification of sternal dehiscence

Type 1:   2–3 days post surgical

            Serosanguinous discharge, negative cultures

            No cellulitis, osteomyelitis or costochondritis

            Debride, re-wire cover with ABx

Type 2:   2–3 weeks post surgical

            Purulent discharge, cellulitis with positive wound cultures

            Underlying osteomyelitis/costochondritis

            Thorough debridement, remove wires, VAC, vascularised tissue cover

Type 3:   2–3 years post surgical

            Chronic discharging sinus

            Positive wound culture

            Condritis and osteomyelitis

            Treat as for a stage 2

Waterlow score for pressure risk

- *Score of > 10 indicates a risk of sore, consider special mattress etc…*

Categories

Body build   Average, below, above

Skin type   Healthy, thin, oedematous, broken

Sex and age

Continence

Mobility

Appetite

Special risks   Tissue malnutrition

                Neurological deficit

                Major surgery/trauma

                Medication

National Pressure Ulcer Advisory Panel Grading System

Grade 1: Non-blanchable erythema of intact skin

Grade 2: Partial thickness skin loss effecting epidermis and dermis

Grade 3: Full-thickness skin loss down to but not involving deep fascia

Grade 4: Full-thickness injury including underlying fascia, bone muscle involved

Hand

Boutonniere deformity classification by Nalebuff

Stage 1: Deformity which is passively correctable. Only 10–15° lag in extension

Full extension of PIPJ may limit DIPJ flexion (tight lateral bands)

Stage 2: Deformity is passively correctable. Flexion deformity starts to give a function loss with MCPJ and DIPJ hyperextension

Stage 3: PIPJ cannot be extended passively

Swan neck deformity classification by Nalebuff

Type 1: Deformity with no loss of motion

Type 2: Deformity with loss of motion at different positions in the MCPJ

Type 3: Deformity with LOM in all MCPJ positions

Type 4: As a type 3 with x-ray changes

Larsens grading of rheumatoid arthritis

0   Normal

1   Osteoporosis, soft tissue swelling

2   Bony erosions, normal architecture maintained

3   Bony erosions, signs of architectural changes

4   Severe joint destruction but joint line is visible

5   Arthritis mutilans with no joint line

Trigger finger classification

Type 1: Pain and nodularity

Type 2: Triggering but self-correctable

Type 3: Triggering correctable manually

Type 4: Locked digit

Mayfield classification of progressive perilunate instability

• *Most common carpal instability occurs between scaphoid and lunate*

Stage 1:   Injury to scapholunate interosseous ligament – scapholunate diastasis

Stage 2:   Further injury causing dorsal subluxation of the capitate relative to lunate

Stage 3:   Perilunate dislocation

Stage 4:   Dislocation of the lunate from the radiolunate fossa

Classification of thumb deformity on RA – Nalebuff

Group 1   Boutonniere with a flexed MCPJ

Group 2   Flexed MCPJ with metacarpal adduction

Group 3   Z thumb, zig-zag thumb or swan-neck def. CMCJ+IP flexed, MCPJ hyper-extended

Group 4   Gamekeeper's thumb

Lispcomb's classification of Volkmann's contracture

Mild: No nerve deficit, muscles tight/short – flexor slide

Moderate: No nerve deficit, some functional muscle loss – flexor slide

Severe: Nerve deficit with little functional muscle. Resection, neurolysis, transfers

V Severe: No motor or sensory activity. Free functional muscle?

Classification of mallet finger deformities (Doyle 1993)

Type 1 :   Closed. Loss of tendon continuity +/– small fragment

Type 2 :   Laceration of skin and tendon at or proximal to DIPJ

Type 3 :   Deep abrasion at DIPJ resulting in loss of continuity

Type 4A :   Transepiphyseal in children

Type 4B :   Fracture 20–50% of articular surface

Type 4C :   Fracture > 50% articular surface and volar subluxation

Leddy and Packer classification of FDP avulsion 1977

Type 1:   Tendon avulsion into the palm. No blood supply

Type 2:   Tendon avulsion +/– bone fragment caught at PIPJ

Type 3:   Bone fragment caught at DIPJ. All vinculae preserved

Type 4:   *Not originally described. Type 1 injury with bone fragment destroying annular and cruciate pulleys on its way to palm*

Urbaniak classification of ring avulsions

Type 1:   Laceration, vascularity intact
Type 2:   Circulation compromised needs revasc, no # or
              dislocation
Type 2A: As above only arterial injury
Type 3:   Total degloving/with or without #/dislocation

Kay modification of Urbaniak, *JHS*, 1989

I   Circulation adequate, with or without skeletal injury
II   Circulation inadequate, with or without skeletal
              injury
IIA   Arterial circulation inadequate only
IIB   Venous circulation inadequate only
III   Circulation inadequate, with fracture or joint injury
IIIA   Arterial circulation inadequate only
IIIB   Venous circulation inadequate only
IV   Complete amputation

Kanavel's 4 cardinal signs

- Fusiform swelling of finger
- Semi-flexed finger position
- Tenderness over flexor sheath
- Pain on passive extension

Weiss and Hastings classification of intra-articular phalangeal fractures

- Oblique palmar
- Long sagittal
- Dorsal coronal
- Palmar coronal

Kienbock's disease (Lichtman et al., *JHS*, 1982)

I   No radiological changes – bone scan hot
II   Increased density but normal shape; minor radial height loss
IIIA   Collapase and sclerosis with carpal disruption. Normal
        scaphoid orientation
IIIB   Scaphoid rotated
IV   Generalized intercarpal arthritis

Salter Harris

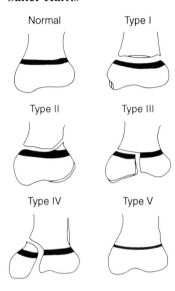

Normal   Type I

Type II   Type III

Type IV   Type V

Type I: Transverse fracture through growth plate
Type II: A fracture through the metaphysic extending through
            the growth plate but sparing the epiphysis (Commonest
            configuration approx 70%)
Type III: A fracture through the epiphysis and growth plate sparing
            the metaphysic
Type IV: A fracture through both the metaphysic, epiphysis and
            growth plate (Next commonest)
Type V: A compression fracture of the growth plate

NB: Types VI–IX described but not commonly used

Reconstruction/Flaps

Fasciocutaneous flap classification – Cormack and Lamberty

Type A: Multiple fasciocutaneous perforators at flap base,
            orientated along the flap's long axis
Type B: Single fasciocutaneous perforator with or without the deep
            artery

Type C: Multiple perforators reaching the fascia from the deep
           artery via the fascial septum – must keep the deep artery
           with the flap. RFF

Type D: As for TC with muscle +/– bone

Mathes and Nahai muscle flap classification by Blood Supply 1981

Type 1:   1 pedicle
           e.g., TFL

Type 2:   1 Major pedicle with other minor pedicles
           e.g., Gracilis

Type 3:   2 dominant pedicles
           e.g., RA, Gluteus maximus

Type 4:   Many segmental pedicles none of which are able to
           completely perfuse
           e.g., Sartorius

Type 5:   1 dominant pedicle with minor pedicles able to supply the
           entire muscle
           e.g., LD

Thatte and Thatte classification of venous flaps

Veno-venous: Unipedicle
                   Bi-pedicled

Arteriovenous: Arteriovenous shunt
                   Arterialized venous flow-through flap

FLAPS

(Anatomy, pedicle, landmarks, dimensions)

Radial forearm

Type C or D

Song, 1982, *Clincs in Plastic Surgery*

A – Radial artery, type C/D, intermuscular septum between
    brachioradialis/FCR distally and PT/brachioradialis
    proximally, superficial to FDS, ulnar to superficial branch
    of radial nerve

P – 20 cm × 2.5 mm

L – mid-point cubital fossa to radial pulse at wrist

D – upto 10 × 40; 4 × 6 can close V to Y

Posterior interosseus artery flap
Masquelat, 1987, *Ann Chir Main*
A – Posterior interosseous A (off common interosseous off ulnar) emerges beneath supinator 6 cm distal to lat. epicondyle; runs in intramuscular septum between extensor compartment 5(EDM) and 6 (ECU)
P – Perforators of PIA; prox. 1/3 0.9–2.7 mm; distal 1/3 0.2–1.2 mm
L – Lateral epicondyle to DRUJ; skin paddle at junction of proximal and middle 1/3. Pivot point 2 cm prox to DRUJ
D – Close direct if <4 cm in width; otherwise SSG. Rise from 6 cm distal to elbow to 4 cm prox to wrist; subcutaneous border of ulnar to radial border of radius

"2656" flap-   2 cm prox to DRUJ
                 6 cm distal to elbow for main perforator
                 5/6 – between compt 5 and 6

Use proximal pedicle if being used free (much larger). 5% no communication with AIA

Lateral arm flap
Katsaros, 1984, *Ann Plast Surg*
A – Posterior collateral radial artery, branch of profunda brachii. Runs between lat. head of triceps and brachialis. Radial nerve anterior to it in spiral groove
P – Septal perforators. 4–8 cm long, 1.5–2.5 mm. Venae comitantes 2.5 mm. Nerve – Posterior brachial cutaneous nerve
L – Deltoid insertion to lat. epicondyle. Skin paddle over distal 1/3 over lateral intermuscular septum
D – 10–14 cm wide (6 cm for direct closure). From midpoint of humerus to 5 cm distal to lateral epicondyle. Can take bone

Pectoralis major
Type V
Ariyan, 1979, *PRS*
A – Pectoral branch of thoraco-acromial trunk. Enters muscle deep where line of junction of middle and lateral thirds of clavicle bisects acromio-xiphisternal line

P – 1. Pec branch of thoraco-acromial trunk; 4 cm long, 2.0 mm wide

2. 1–6th intercostal cutaneous perforators of internal mammary artery

L – Acromial-xiphis. line bisection with junction middle and lateral one-third of clavicle. Skin paddle either medial or in IMF

D 15 × 20 cm

Fibula

Type C/D

Taylor, 1975, *PRS*

Hidalgo, 1989, *PRS*

A – Peroneal artery sends in nutrient branch 16 cm below fibular head. Skin paddle supplied by cutaneous perforators in posterior intermuscular septum

P – 4 cm, 0.2 mm. Can be lengthened with periosteal dissection

L – Skin paddle on line from head of fibula to posterior border of lat. Malleolus, centred on junction of middle and distal thirds

D – Bone up to 26 cm

Skin up to 8 × 15 cm

Medial Plantar Artery

Myamato, 1987, *PRS*

Type B

A – Medial plantar artery, terminal branch of post. tibial artery; runs between Ab Hall and FDB bellies. Perforators supply skin paddle on medial edge of central plantar fascia.

P – 12 cm × 1.5 mm

L – Skin paddle on instep along line between head of 1st MT and midpoint of heel, over Ab Hall muscle. Do not transgress onto weight bearing areas of the foot.

D – 6 × 12 cm

Tensor fascia lata

Hill, 1978, *PRS*

Type I

A – Transverse branch of lateral circumflex femoral artery from profunda femoris. Divides into 3 and supplies muscle in thirds. 5–7 musculocutaneous perforators supply skin paddle, extends to 5 cm above knee.

P – 6 cm × 2.0 mm

L – Axis runs along anterior edge of muscle in line from ASIS to lateral tibial condyle. Pedicle enters 6–10 cm from ASIS on the line. Muscle 3 cm wide, 15 cm long.

D – 10 × 20 cm for direct closure, 20 × 40 cm with SSG

Anterolateral thigh

Song, 1984, *Br J Plast Surg*

Type B/C

A – Perforators from descending branch lateral circumflex femoral artery. Approx. 80% musculocutaneous, 20% septocutaneous either through vastus lateralis or in septum between it and rectus femoris. 2–3 main perforators

P – 12 cm × 2.0 mm

L – Axis is line from ASIS to lateral border of patella. Perforator tends to be in a quadrant 3 cm postero-distal to the midpoint of this line

D – 10 × 20 cm for direct closure, 15 × 35 cm with SSG

Gracilis

Harii, 1976, *PRS*

McGraw, 1976, *PRS*

Type II

A – Terminal branch of medial circumflex femoral artery from profunda femoris. Enters muscle 10 cm inferior to pubic tubercle

P – 7 cm × 1.5 mm

L – Axis is 2 cm posterior to line from pubic tubercle to medial femoral condyle. Main cutaneous perforator at about 10 cm from pubic tubercle, where the vessel enters the muscle

D – Muscle 6 × 30 cm. Skin 8 × 15 cm

Trauma

Mangled Extremity Severity Score (MESS) (Johansen et al.; *J Trauma*; 1984)
Scores of 7+ predictive of amputation

Soft tissue/skeletal injury
   Low – very high energy injury. *Score 1–4*
Limb ischaemia
   Reduced pulse with normal perfusion – cool paralysed numb. *Score 1–3*. Doubled if
   ischaemia time > 6 h
Shock
   Systolic BP always > 90 mmHg – persistent hypotension. *Score 0–2*
Age
   <30, 30–50, 50+. *Score 0–2*

Classification of open tibial fractures, Gustillo and Anderson; *J Trauma*; 1986

Type 1:	Wound < 1 cm
Type 2:	Wound > 1 cm without extensive soft tissue injury, flaps and avulsions
Type 3A:	Adequate soft tissue cover in a tibial fracture despite extensive soft-tissue damage or high-energy trauma
Type 3B:	Extensive soft tissue loss with periosteal stripping and bone exposure. May be heavily contaminated
Type 3C:	Open fracture with associated arterial injury requiring repair

Byrd and Spicer classification of open tibial fractures (*PRS*; 1985)

Type 1:	Low energy spiral/oblique fracture clean <2 cm wound
Type 2:	Moderate energy, comminuted or displaced fracture >2 cm laceration, muscle contusion but no non-viable muscle
Type 3:	High energy – extensive soft tissue, skin and muscle loss
Type 4:	Extreme energy resulting in degloving, crush or vascular injury

Incidences

Hypospadia	1/300	2,000 lb/per annum UK
Positional plagiocephaly	1/300	
Cleft lip/palate	1/600–700	1,000 lb/per annum UK
Syndactyly	1/1,000–3,000	
Submucosal cleft palate	1/1,000	
Neurofibromatosis	1/3,000	
Hemifacial microsomy	1/5,000	
Anotia	1/6,000 UK, 1/4,000 Japan, 1/1,000 Native American	
Constriction Ring Syndrome	1/15,000	
Crouzon	1/15–25,000	
Poland	1/25,000	
Facial cleft	1/25,000	
Treacher-Collins	1/25–50,000	
Craniosynostosis	1/25,000	
Gorlins	1/60–150,000	
Aperts	1/160,000	
Exstrophy	1/60,000	
Xeroderma pigmentosum	1/million	
BCC		650/100,000
SCC		150/100,000
MM		6–10/100,000
Sarcoma		25/100,000

Other Useful Bits for Exams

Aeitiology of synostosis

- Virchow suggested a primary sutural abnormality
- McCarthy a dural abnormality
- Moss an abnormality in the skull base
- Recently FGFR abnormalities have been discovered in some synostosis

Diagnostic criteria for RA (American College of Rheumatology)

Morning stiffness
Arthritis of 3 or more joint areas
Arthritis of hand joints
Symmetric arthritis

The above should be present for 6 weeks

Rheumatoid nodules
RHF +ve
X-Ray changes
- 4 or more indicate RA
- Operate proximal to distal with the exception of the PIPJ boutonniere where PIPJ function effects MCPJ

DVT
Risk groups

Low	Minor surgery <30 min. Any age. No risk factors
	Major surgery >30 min. Age <40. No other risk factors
	Minor trauma or medical illness
Moderate	Major surgery. Age ?40 or other risk factors
	Major medical illness: heart/lung disease, CA, inflammatory bowel disease
	Major trauma/burns
	Minor surgery, trauma, medical illness in pt. with previous DVT, PE or thrombophilia
High	Major orthopaedic surgery or # pelvis, hip, lower limb
	Major abdo/pelvic surgery for ca
	Major surgery, trauma, medical illness in pt with DVT, PE or thrombophilia
	Lower limb paralysis (e.g., stroke, paraplegia)
	Major lower limb amputation

DVT/Thromboembolism risk factors

Patient	Disease
Age	Trauma or surgery, esp. pelvis, hip, lower limb
Obesity	Malignancy, esp. pelvic, abdominal metastatic
Immobility	Heart failure

Patient	Disease
Pregnancy/ puerperium	Recent M I
High dose oestrogen therapy	Lower limb paralysis
Prev. DVT/PE	Infection
Thrombophilia	Inflammatory bowel disease
	Nephrotic syndrome
	Polycythaemia
	Paraproteinaemia
	Paroxysmal nocturnal haemoglobinuria
	Behcet's disease
	Homocystinaemia

High risk	1. Graduated elastic anti-embolism stockings (e.g., Kendal T.E.D.) plus
	2. Low molecular weight heparin (contact hospital pharmacy for available products and dose)
	or
	Adjusted dose warfarin (INR 2–3)
	3. Consider intermittent pneumatic compression
Moderate risk	1. Graduated elastic anti-embolism stockings (e.g., Kendal T.E.D.)
	and/or
	2. Low molecular weight heparin (contact hospital pharmacy for available products and dose)
Low risk	1. Early mobilisation

Foetal wound healing

- Less inflammation
- More collagen type 3
- Epithelialisation more rapid
- Angiogenesis is reduced
- Collagen deposition rapid, not excessive and organised
- In first trimester may be scarless i.e. regenerative

First and second set phenomenon – Gibson and Medawar rejection

- Reaction to allograft such as skin on first exposure
  - 1–3 days graft takes as per usual
  - 4–7 days infiltration with leucocytes and thrombi with punctate haemorrhages evident
  - 7–9 days blood flow ceases and graft undergoes necrosis
- Second set phenomenon occurs if host is exposed to allogenic material from the same source again
  - Immediate hyperacute rejection
  - Graft does not undergo any revascularisation
- Graft destruction is by both
  - Direct destruction mediated by the cellular system CD4/8 T-cells
  - Indirect mediated by humoral system. Stimulated B lymphocytes produce an antibody which binds with the antigen and stimulates the destruction via complement
- HLAs A B and DR are most important mediators of tissue rejection (Class 1 and 2)

Features of raised ICP

- Tense fontanelles
- Irratibility
- Seizures
- Papilloedema
- Psychomotor retardation

Glasgow Coma Scale 3–15

	1	2	3	4	5	6
Eyes	Does not open eyes	Opens eyes in response to painful stimuli	Opens eyes in response to voice	Opens eyes spontaneously	N/A	N/A
Verbal	Makes no sounds	Incomprehensible sounds	Utters inappropriate words	Confused, disoriented	Oriented, converses normally	N/A
Motor	Makes no movements	Extension to painful stimuli decerebrate response	Abnormal flexion to painful stimuli decorticate response	Flexion/ withdrawal to painful stimuli	Localizes painful stimuli	Obeys commands

Huger's zones of blood supply – Anterior abdominal wall 1979

Zone 1:   Mid abdomen supplied by deep epigastric arcade

Zone 2:   Lower abdomen supplied by epigastric arcade and external iliac. Superficial to the fascia is provided by SIEA and SEPA, both from the femoral

Zone 3:   Lateral abdomen and flanks. Blood supply from the intercostals, subcostal and lumbar arteries. Intercostals enter the abdomen between transverses and internal oblique and anastamose with SEA and DIEA

Infection preventing SSG taking

- 10^5 organisms per gram

Nerve types

- Group A
  - Alpha – Motor and proprioceptive
  - Beta – Pressure and proprioceptive
  - Gamma – Motor to muscle spindles
  - Delta – Touch, pain and temperature
- Group B – Myelinated pre-ganglionic autonomic nerves
- Group C – Myelinated post-ganglionic autonomic nerves

Radiological changes in OA

- Joint space narrowing
- Sclerosis of the bones
- Bone cysts
- Spurs, osteophytes, exostoses

Scoring systems for Inhalational Injury

- Many tried
- Aim to predict outcome
- Based on PaO2/FiO2 ratio, chest x-ray, peek inspiratory pressures and bronchoscopy
- Brown and Warden
- Kansella

Suture material

- Absorbable
    - Catgut
        - Submucosal sheep intestine
        - Strength lost at 10 days lasts a month
    - Polyglycolic acid – Dexon
        - Hydrolysed
        - Loses strength at 21 days and absorbed at 90
    - Polyglactin 910 – Vicryl
        - Loses strength at 21 days and absorbed at 90
        - Synthetic braided suture
    - Polyglecaprone 25 – Monocryl
        - Loses strength at 21 days and absorbed at 90
    - Polydioxanone – PDS
        - Loses strength at 3 months and absorbed at 6 months
- Non-absorbable
    - Silk
    - Polyamide – Nylon
    - Polypropylene – Prolene
    - Stainless steel

UV light wavelengths

- UVA: 320–400 nm
- UVB: 280–320 nm
- UVC: 200–280 nm

Index

S. Hettiaratchy et al. (eds.), *Plastic Surgery*,
DOI 10.1007/978-1-84882-116-3,
© Springer-Verlag London Limited 2012